"TRANSPLANT is a compulsive pleasure.
Brilliant heart surgeon Athan Carras is in midlife
crisis and is tempted by a ruthless billionaire to do
the unthinkable. Seduction becomes coercion in this
fast-paced thriller that cuts to core questions of ethics
in modern medicine."

Robert Picardo
Emergency Medical Hologram (EMH)
also known as The Doctor, Star Trek: Voyager

"Heart-rending, intriguing medical mystery. The
most difficult challenges in medical care are not the result of technical advances, they are the result of the intense human commitments and moral
dilemmas that these advances make possible."

Harold W. Baillie, Provost, University of Scranton

"A gripping tale of violence and intrigue
set within the world of transplant surgery, Dr. Elefteriades makes abstract
ethical questions about life and death bristle with urgency. This is a skilled
and accurate depiction of heart transplant and a horrifying scenario that
could occur when money and power join forces."

Mariell Jessup MD
Professor of Medicine
Director, Heart Failure/Transplant program
University of Pennsylvania

"If you are looking for **a rip-roaring thriller,** stop. You've found
it. Transplant has enough gritty background detail to make it entirely convincing and more than enough action and pace to keep you glued to it."

Dave Duncan, author of *The Alchemist's Pursuit.*

Transplant

A novel by
John A. Elefteriades, MD

Robot
Binaries
&Press

Transplant

PUBLISHED BY ROBOT BINARIES & PRESS CORP
704 Spadina Avenue, #134, Toronto, Ontario M5S 2S9

Book and cover design by Kathy Harestad   www.kathyart.com

This book is a work of fiction. It should not be used as the basis for any medical decision. Please check with your health-care provider before making any health-care decision.

Library and Archives Canada Cataloguing in Publication
Elefteriades, John A.
    Transplant / John A. Elefteriades.
ISBN 978-1-894689-10-6
    I. Title.

PS3605.L43T73 2009   813'.6   C2008-905841-0

Transplant

Chapter 1

Doctor, I cannot forbid you to perform that procedure," said the clipped, nasal voice in Athan Carras's ear, "but I emphatically withhold the permission you are seeking from the committee."

You vindictive son of a bitch, Carras thought, but into the phone he said, "You don't have that authority, doctor. You are just the vice-chair of the Human Investigations Committee. Only the chairman has the right to grant or withhold approval."

There was a silence on the line, then Carras could hear the thin smile in Dr. James Bonar Auldfield's voice when he said, "You should have read the committee's terms of reference more closely, doctor. In the absence of Dr. Bentham, all of his powers devolve to me."

"For God's sake," Carras said, "that's Cory Goldenberg on my operating table. Leave aside that he's a friend and colleague of both of us, he's one of the top cardiologists in the world. If the technique works, he could live another ten years, save hundreds of lives. But if I don't do it, he'll be dead before morning. Guaranteed."

Auldfield's voice was bright with a cold glee. "I've told you, doctor, it's entirely your decision," he said. "You agreed that there will be no human experimentation until the HIC has seen long-term results from the animal trials. However, if you want to disavow the covenant you have made with the committee, you are free to break your word."

"But you won't cut me an inch of slack, will you, Boner?"

Carras heard the sniff that preceded Auldfield's final remark. "I must do as my conscience dictates. You do as you wish." There was a click and the line was dead.

Shouldn't have called him Boner, Carras thought. Auldfield hated the nickname he'd acquired when they'd been students together. But Carras realized it wouldn't have made any difference if he'd abased himself to flatter the other man's delicate ego.

Back in Operating Room 15 of Yale Medical Center, Craig Mason looked up from the dials of the heart-lung machine that was keeping Cory Goldenberg from sliding into death and said, "Are we go?"

Carras took up his customary place on the patient's left and swept his gaze over the monitors before answering. "Bentham's on some kind of retreat in Montana. Left his cell at home. Can't be reached before the end of the week."

"So who's on deck for him?" Mason said, then his eyes widened as he answered the question for himself. "Oh, fuck me. Boner, right?"

Carras sighed. "And Boner says we're on our own."

"Well fuck him with the broomstick he rode in on," said Mason. "Like I'm going to let Cory die because that little piss-ant thinks he's Pontius Pilate? Let's do this, Ath. Now."

"Let me think."

• • •

Cory Goldenberg should have known better. Although he was a senior cardiologist with Harvard Medical School, he suffered from a condition known as aortic regurgitation: a weakness in his heart's outflow valve that did not let it be a one-way-only door. After expelling all the blood in the left ventricle, it didn't slam shut and stay tight; instead, the valve let a little blood leak back into the heart. The result was a progressive weakening of the organ.

Any heart surgeon knew the answer to aortic regurgitation: cut out the faulty natural valve and put in an artificial one. These days it was a routine procedure and post-operative complications were next to nil. Goldenberg could have had his operation any time over the several years since the onset of his condition.

But Goldenberg was a conservative cardiologist. He had taught for years that surgery should not be an instant resort. Patients should wait until there was definite evidence that the heart was enlarging. With hearts, bigger is not better; bigger is certainly not stronger—an enlarged heart is a weak heart. Goldenberg taught that until enlargement was evident, surgery should be put off, and he practiced what he preached.

In the meantime, he drove himself to a high level of fitness. He played tennis every day, between morning rounds and afternoon office hours, often taking on much younger opponents and beating them in straight sets. He rode a bike and trained with light weights. At sixty, he was lean, strong and looked fit.

"I've started to enlarge," he had said, sitting in Carras's long, shoe box-shaped office in Yale's venerable Farnum Building, between the modern medical center and the old red-brick morgue. They looked at the echocardiographic images from the lab. The enlargement was small—only one centimeter in diameter—but noticeable.

"No point waiting," Carras said. "We'll perform the procedure tomorrow morning." He looked again at the echo results and said, "I wish you hadn't waited."

It was an argument as old as modern surgery. Clinicians like Goldenberg preferred to use non-invasive therapies—drugs, exercise, change of diet—to treat the myriad afflictions that the human body is at risk of. Surgeons opted to isolate the part at fault and if they couldn't repair or replace it, they'd cut it out altogether and let the body's systems adapt.

The body was designed with built-in redundancy. Life could go on without a gall bladder or a spleen, with only one lung or kidney or with substantial portions of the liver missing. But humans were issued only one heart and it had to last a lifetime, and Carras felt there was no point in unduly stressing the organ when a quick and simple surgical repair could avoid trouble.

Goldenberg thought surgery was inherently dangerous, even under gifted hands. A certain number of patients who went under anesthesia never came out of it—the fraction was tiny, but that didn't make any difference when relatives arrived at the hospital to visit Uncle Waldo after his minor knee surgery and found him chilling in the morgue.

"You're more likely to be hit by lightning," Carras said. "Or bitten by a shark."

"If I stay in during lightning storms and stay out of shark-infested waters, the chances of being hit or bit are zero," Goldenberg answered. "As are my chances of dying on an operating table if I stay off one."

"You won't die on mine," Carras said.

"Sometimes I wonder about you, Ath," Goldenberg said. "It's as if you see yourself in a head-to-head contest with death."

"I wouldn't put it so dramatically," Carras said.

"Maybe not out loud," the cardiologist agreed, "but I wonder if there are times when you look across the operating table and see the old reaper reaching for your patient, and then it's not about the patient any more. It's about winning."

"All right, sometimes I do feel defeated when I lose a patient. And I hate it. Don't we all?"

"Sure, to some extent," Goldenberg said. "Just don't let it get too personal. Even when you're operating on me. Remember, doctor, pride goeth before a fall."

"I'm not the one who's waited until his heart's enlarged, doctor," Carras said. "That looks to be a fair-sized stumble on your part."

"Touché," said the clinician, "but a little below the belt, don't you think?"

For a moment, Carras was tempted to say, *Sorry, that was a low blow.* But he and Cory had argued over similar cases so many times, in print and face to face at conferences, that the combative habit just naturally came to the fore. And when in combat mode, Athan Carras did not say sorry. *Besides*, he told himself, *an apology's not what Cory needs. He needs his heart fixed.*

Carras fixed it the next morning, in an operation that was entirely routine from Goldenberg's first shot of sedative to the post-op visit by Carras in the intensive care unit. The new pyrolite carbon valve was clicking away in the cardiologist's chest and blood flow was normal. But would the moderately enlarged heart recover and return to normal?

It took five years for the definitive answer to come in. Cory Goldenberg's heart had not recovered. Weakened, it had continued to grow larger and less powerful. Partly through medication but mostly by sheer will power, the clinician had been able to carry on with his teaching and practice, but his condition deteriorated, at first slowly then later at an accelerated pace. Now, at sixty-five, he was suffering from end-stage heart failure; the enlargement and contractile weakness of his left ventricle were so extreme that the eleven different medications he took each day could not compensate. He came to Carras for a transplant.

The choice of a Yale surgeon by a prominent Harvard physician prompted some ironic comments in Ivy League circles. Carras had held his own in many a contentious academic debate, sometimes supplementing scientific fact with acid wit. He was not universally loved by his peers, of whom there were relatively few, and some of those he had bested detested him.

But as Goldenberg said in a widely reposted e-mail, "Sure, Carras can be arrogant, but he has every right to be. In my case, he was right and I was wrong, and if I come out of this alive it's because of him."

The wait for a suitable donor heart stretched into weeks, then into months. Goldenberg was maintained on a continuous infusion of the drug dobutamine, which artificially strengthened his heartbeat and maintained an adequate outflow of blood from his failing left ventricle. The cardiotonic medication was delivered to his heart by a catheter connected to a pump. Some days, he used Carras's office to work on a paper he was writing for the American Journal of Cardiologists.

Goldenberg was at Carras's desk when he finally collapsed from pulmonary edema—he began to drown from backing up of blood and pressure into his lungs. Fortunately, Carras's secretary, Karen Ferguson, was keeping an eye on him and within minutes she had arranged for the cardiologist to be wheeled up the long glassed-in walkway between the Farnum Building and the recently built medical center's coronary care unit. He was placed on a ventilator that sent high-flow oxygen into his bloodstream, the enriched mixture making up for poor blood flow from his weakened heart.

Two days later, they found a suitable donor heart. In Boston, a fifteen-year-old boy had discovered where his father had hidden the ignition key of his Yamaha 650 motorcycle and decided to take the bike out for a spin. Helmetless, leaning so far over that one knee almost touched the asphalt, the boy swept around a blind curve and smashed into an oil delivery truck. The surgeons at Boston General kept him technically alive for eleven hours while they assessed the neurological implications of his massive head injury, but the victim was brain dead.

The boy was big for his age and had been a good athlete. His blood type was a match for Goldenberg's. When the Yale donor team flew by Lear jet to Boston and harvested the heart, the organ looked perfect. They also took a lymph node for tissue typing and the lab result was phoned through to Yale while the jet was carrying the team and the heart back to New Haven.

It was two a.m. when Carras heard they had a good match. He ordered Goldenberg prepped and transferred to OR 15, his favorite of the medical center's five cardiothoracic operating suites. The heart arrived on time, safe in its zip-lock bag of saline solution resting on a bed of ice in a cooler that would not have looked out of place on a picnic blanket—except for the large blue cross and the lettering that said HUMAN ORGAN—DO NOT TOUCH.

The operating team opened the patient's chest and began to place the catheters that would allow them to connect to the heart lung machine. The systolic pressure in Cory Goldenberg's arteries was a limp 85 over 40, well below normal readings of 120 over 80. That was as expected. The problem came when the catheter in the pulmonary artery reported pressure of 70 over 40 in the cardiologist's lungs, way above the 25/10 pressure that would have been a normal.

"We've got pulmonary hypertension," Carras said.

On the other side of the table, Craig Mason said, "How bad?" and when he saw the numbers on the monitor, "Oh, shit."

Now a heart transplant could not guarantee the life of Cory Goldenberg. Years of progressive heart disease had thickened and scarred the blood vessels in the cardiologist's lungs. Even a heart from a young, healthy fifteen-year-old might not have the strength to overcome the vessels' acquired resistance.

Now that immunosuppressive drugs had overcome the problems of rejection of foreign tissue by a recipient's immune system, pulmonary hypertension was the leading cause of death after heart transplants. The normal heart was put into a system that had adapted to abnormality. The normal heart often couldn't handle the load. Fifty per cent of such patients died not long after receiving new hearts. Cory Goldenberg's numbers put him in the highest category of risk.

The right ventricle of the donor's heart had only had to cope with normal systolic pressure in the maze of blood vessels that permeated the teenager's lungs. It was, as is natural, a thin-walled chamber, only one fifth the thickness of the powerful left ventricle, which had to pump blood to the rest of the body.

But the right side of Cory Goldenberg's heart had spent almost the same number of years pushing against blood that had backed up in his lungs because the weakened left side of the organ could not pull it along into the rest of the circulatory system with sufficient strength. To compensate, the right side of Goldenberg's diseased heart had grown unnaturally thick and strong.

Carras had lectured on the problem often enough. "The right side of the diseased heart is like a body builder who has been curling fifty and sixty pound weights, building Schwarzenegger biceps. That's the kind of muscle it takes to force blood into the congested lungs.

"But the normal heart is Joe Average, used to curling maybe twenty pounds. Now we put that heart into the chest of someone with serious pulmonary hypertension, and it's like handing an ordinary person a great big dumbbell and saying, 'Here, curl this. And keep curling it all day, and all day tomorrow and forever.'"

Carras had not only been lecturing on the problem, however; he had the kind of mind that, when faced with no as the answer to a scientific problem, shot back with *why the hell not?*

Cutting out a heart that had an unnaturally strong right ventricle and a desperately weak left one, and putting in an organ that was normal on both sides, simply didn't work. There had to be another way, yet every logical approach he considered came up dry. But Carras had learned that when his rational mind had gone round and round a problem and found no logical answer, sometimes his unconscious would pull in a solution from way out of any conventional orbit. One of those wild surmises came to Carras one night as he lay dreaming.

He was in the old family kitchen, in the house on Philadelphia's Market Street where he had grown up. He took a loaf of bread out of the zinc lined drawer underneath the counter, but when he went to cut a slice from it, he saw that one end was covered in mold. He carried the loaf to the trash container under the sink and was going to throw it away, but then his father was there, young and dark-mustached as he'd been when Athan was a boy, wearing the stained coveralls from the service station that he owned.

He took the bread from Carras's hand, put it back on the counter and sliced it in half. The moldy end he threw into the trash bin; the other half he held out to Carras, saying in Greek, *"To miso eine kalo."* The half is good.

Carras came up out of the dream with the words still echoing in his mind. It was either a dumb idea or it was brilliant. Instead of removing the whole heart, why not take out only the diseased left side and sew the new organ to the Schwarzenegger half that remained? The patient would have a heart-and-a-half, with two right ventricles to cope with the overly high ambient pressure in the lungs.

On the face of it, it was a wacko proposition. The heart was one mass of specialized cardiac muscle. No one had ever tried to separate the two halves. Even in folklore, a broken heart was fatal. How could he cut out half a heart then stitch a foreign organ to what was left? Carras didn't know, but once the idea took him he had to find out.

He put together a small team, him and Craig Mason plus some students and residents to assist. They started in the morgue, cutting and pasting the hearts of cadavers. Then they sought research funding and began experimenting with live animals.

Their research plan had estimated two or three years to develop the heart-and-a-half procedure or to prove that it was impossible. In the end, it was five years of part-time lab work. There were endless problems: bleeding from the cut edges of cardiac muscle after they were sutured to each other; interruption of the flow of nutrients to the heart's muscle cells, so that they starved and died; interference with the network of nerves that acted as the heart's internal pacemaker.

One after another, they faced the problems and solved them, until they could perform every aspect of the new operation routinely, efficiently and consistently. There came a day when Carras and Mason could say to each other with a confidence born of experience, "We could do this with a human being."

Could, however, was not the same as should. Mason was ready to proceed immediately to a human trial. There were patients whose lives might depend on it. But Carras was not ready.

"Horseshit and hellfire," Mason said, "it was your damn dream started this. Listen to your unconscious and let's schedule the first op."

They were in the lab watching a pig that now had a heart and a half munch its way through a cabbage. The animal's chest incision was almost fully healed.

"Look at Porky, here," Mason said. "He's happy as a pig in shit. There's people need this special thing we can do."

"Human trials are a big risk," Carras said. "Animal models aren't always a reliable indicator."

"Well, what do you want to do? We don't have any half-man-half-animals to work our way up through."

"Let's take it to the HIC," Carras said. "I talked to Charlie Vance and he said they'd be willing to assume responsibility for oversight."

Carras's long-time friend Charlie Vance was a dual degree holder, with an MD and a PhD in philosophy, who specialized in medical ethics—he described himself as a "doctor of philosophy and a philosopher of doctoring." Vance was a member of Yale's multidisciplinary Human Investigations Committee, whose purpose was to guide and regulate researchers through the complex thickets of moral questions that often sprang up between the orderly gardens of existing knowledge and the deep dark woods that were the unknown.

The committee met in the august Beaumont Room above the rotunda of the massive Sterling Library. Carras and Mason presented a summary of their work to date, much of it already familiar to the committee members from papers the two researchers had published in professional journals. "We are confident that we have validated the technique in the animal models and believe it is time to consider a human trial," Carras concluded the presentation.

The committee's chair, the renowned geneticist Taylor Bentham, looked to his left and right, peering over his half-glasses at the other HIC members ranged on either side of him behind the long antique table. "Responses?" he said.

Charlie Vance had always reminded Carras of Jack Nicholson playing Mr. Chips: the face was a close resemblance and the voice was almost identical. Now the ethicist leaned forward from one end of the panel and said, "I have complete confidence in Drs. Carras and Mason. It is good of them to have come before us, even though they did not have to. I say we define a set of conditions governing a first human trial and let them get on with it."

Bentham nodded and again looked up and down the table, finding a general sense of agreement with the proposal. Then a nasal voice said, "I'm not as sanguine as Dr. Vance."

"Oh, fuck me sideways," Mason whispered to Carras, "when did Boner get on this committee?"

Carras's only reply was a shrug, his attention focused entirely on Auldfield. "I don't find the animal trials," the small man continued, placing one delicate finger to his slim jaw line, "to be suitably comprehensive."

Vance said, "They've been at it five years."

"The point of this procedure," Auldfield said, "is to overcome the problem of pulmonary hypertension resulting from chronic heart disease. Yet all of the animal subjects have had normal lung and circulatory systems."

"Shit," said Mason. "He's out to ream us."

"No, he's right," said Carras. "We should have thought of that."

"He only thought of it so he could ream us," Mason said.

But Carras was already rising to his feet. "Dr. Auldfield is right. We will test the procedure on animals that have boggy lungs. We can find a way to induce iatrogenic pulmonary hypertension and challenge our operation against it."

They took healthy pigs and injected a caustic drug that engendered a kind of congestion in their lungs that closely mimicked pulmonary hypertension in humans, left the animals in that condition for a few weeks, then performed the new procedure. Each time the new heart-and-a-half began to beat they watched the monitor and saw the enhanced organ steamroller through the high blood pressure in the lungs.

But when they went back to the committee, Auldfield said, "You have an experimental group but no control group. How do we know that an ordinary heart transplant might not have handled the induced lung pressures?"

Mason wanted to argue. "You know that regular transplants don't handle the problem in humans. That's why we came up with this procedure."

But Carras again had to cede Auldfield the ethical high ground. An experiment without a control group proved nothing. So they went back to the lab and did normal heart transplants on pigs with boggy lungs. The normal hearts failed, just as they always had in humans, and the pigs died.

"All very good," said James Bonar Auldfield when they appeared before the committee again, "but how long do your experimental subjects live?"

"What's that got to do with anything?" Mason said. It was normal to sacrifice the experimental animals as soon as the results of the experiments were known. It was difficult to care for the creatures after major surgery, especially larger ones like calves and pigs. It was also expensive. "It's not provided for in our budget," he concluded.

"Are you comfortable performing this procedure on a human subject," Auldfield said, "when you have no indication, even from animal models, what the long-term results will be?"

"He's got us again," Mason whispered to Carras.

"He's right again," Carras replied.

"He just wants to screw us."

"Actually, he wants to screw me," Carras said. "You're just collateral damage."

"Collateral or not, I'm still getting damaged here, Ath," Mason said. "I think we've taken enough of this crap. If we put up a fight, the committee will split but I'll bet Bentham will rule in our favor."

"But we'll have won through politics. Auldfield would have the ethical high ground."

"So what? We can get on with saving some lives," Mason said. "Listen, Ath, what's more important, launching a procedure that can save lives or beating that little prick at his own game?"

But Carras wouldn't budge.

Carras knew that medical ethics had come a long way since the fifties, sixties and seventies, the heyday of creative innovations in cardiac surgery. In those days, the great cardiothoracic pioneers—Cooley, DeBakey and Lillehei—had wasted no time between preliminary testing of a new procedure and the first application to human patients. Many of those patients, even most of them, had died before the surgeons got it right.

Carras had lost patients. Sometimes all his skill and experience couldn't let him undo the harm that disease or trauma can do to a human heart. He remembered every one of the failures, and every one of them hurt.

It was wrong to risk people's lives, even the lives of those already on the lip of death, if there was a way to pretest the procedure on animals. He'd said it often enough in the debates that went on among those who were literally the cutting edge of new medical techniques. Now James Bonar Auldfield was knowingly using Carras's own standards against him.

"He wants to be able to call me a hypocrite," he told Mason, their heads together and voices low. "I'm not going to give him the opportunity."

"Sticks and fucking stones, Ath."

"No, Craig, I'm going to agree to the extended trials."

"But who's going to say when enough time has passed?"

"Bentham's a sound man. When it's been a reasonable length of time, he'll say it's enough."

Mason looked at Auldfield's carefully composed face. "You never should've hung that nickname on the little asshole," he said.

It had been two months and three days since the last series of operations on animals who'd been given boggy lungs. The three pig patients were coming along fine, the enhanced hearts pumping blood into resistant blood vessels that would have stymied normal transplanted organs. The pigs were thriving while human beings with similar problems were being denied heart transplants because of the risk of failure; or worse, they were receiving the transplants and dying.

Carras had decided to give the trials a few more days—that would make it ten weeks—before going back to the committee. Then Cory Goldenberg had collapsed in his office and the Boston teenager's heart had been a good match.

• • •

Carras looked into the gaping space that was the opened chest of Dr. Cory Goldenberg, at the grossly swollen mass that was the cardiologist's diseased heart, its function assumed for now by the humming, gurgling heart-lung machine. *Let me think*, he had said to Mason. But what was there to think about? He knew he could save this useful man.

"Look, Ath," Mason said, "so you gave your word to the committee. Do you think if Bentham was here he'd tell you to plop that kid's heart into Cory and if he died, tough shit?"

"It will be technically a breach of ethics," Carras said.

"Then we're doing it?"

"We're doing it."

"Damn straight," Mason said, and Martini the anesthesiologist put in a "Roger that, Ath."

"But this is on me, guys," Carras said. "If we blow it, Auldfield will call out the dogs. But it's me they'll be chasing, because it's me he wants."

"And we all know why," Mason said, with a wink to one of the nurses.

"Never mind the history," Carras said. He held out his gloved hand to the circulating nurse and said, "Scalpel."

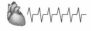

Chapter 2

Even if the event that made them lifelong enemies had never happened, Athan Carras and James Bonar Auldfield would never have been friends. They were as different as two members of the same profession could be. Auldfield was an internist; he treated the body as a unified system of intricately interlocking parts and processes and believed that the physician's role, through precise and minimal intervention, was to help it heal itself.

As a surgeon, Carras was one of the breed that Auldfield disparaged as, "cowboys with scalpels instead of six-guns; cut first and ask questions later."

"Auldfield," Carras once told a colleague, "has misread the first commandment of the ancient Hippocratic Oath. Where it says, *primum non nocere*, or 'First, do no harm,' he thinks it says, *perpetuum ponderare*, or 'Think about it forever.' Auldfield will ponder away until it's too late to do anything at all. That's when he'll call me in to do an operation. We've had patients leave here in the morgue wagon who would've walked out if they hadn't been on Boner's list."

It was a harsh judgment for one doctor to levy upon another, even in a private conversation. The fact that Auldfield had been standing outside Carras's office and heard every word, made the impact worse. The internist was a man who forgave little and forgot nothing.

The root of their enmity went back to their student days, when fate had shown a wicked sense of humor in decreeing that they would be assigned adjoining rooms in Yale's graduate student housing. They were ill-matched neighbors. Despite four years at one of the world's best universities, Carras remained a rough diamond from a side street in Philly, propelled into Yale by a top percentile score in his SATs and a brilliant showing at Lansdowne high school. Auldfield had advanced placidly through the best private schools of New England, in the footsteps of ancestors whose portraits hung on the walls of Yale's oldest halls.

As an undergraduate, Carras had studied French and psychology, his adolescent passions. Auldfield was drawn to computers, which in those days were room-filling machines that calculated by shuffling thousands of cards full of punched holes.

Growing up bilingual had given Carras a facility with languages. His professors were pushing him to continue in French and eventually to teach. Unable to decide, he opted to take all of the graduate school entrance exams— French, law, medicine—and see how he did. The Med exam was first, and he scored so well that, assured of a place in Yale's prestigious medical school, he decided to spare himself the arduous task of taking the other exams.

He could not be said to have had a calling for medicine, but it was interesting enough. It was in his third year that the lightning struck, the first time he assisted at surgery and saw the intricate workings of a human body, the incredible architecture of muscle and bone, the mysterious networks that combine air and liquid and a host of electrochemical triggers in an unfathomable manner that somehow allows what would otherwise be a pile of inert meat to speak and sing, to compose like a Moliére or a Garth Brooks, to paint a Picasso or doodle on a cocktail napkin. From then on, he was hooked.

James Bonar Auldfield followed his own path to the doors of the medical school. Carras doubted the clinician harbored any romantic affection for the human body—it was all by the numbers for Auldfield, and that was why the Ivy League scion had ended up as one of the world's authorities on hemodynamics, the abstruse study of blood-flow patterns and pressures within the heart.

But their differences of background and personality were not enough to make them enemies. They should have been like two parallel species, wildebeest and zebra, sharing the same stretch of veldt, scarcely aware of each other's existence. But then chance put the thinness of a graduate student residence wall between them, through which—while he tried to concentrate on details of mathematical models—Auldfield could hear the clink of bottles and the raucous laughter of Carras's fellow surgeons-to-be.

There were other sounds which bothered Auldfield even more. Young

Athan Carras had a body, face and manner that young women responded to. It was the seventies and the sexual revolution. Carras never noticed his next door neighbor's painful shyness around the opposite sex. Nor did he consider the effects on Auldfield of having to listen to the guy next door plow his way through a succession of willing partners, some of whom loudly expressed their appreciation of crucial moments in unmistakable terms.

But even that would have done no more than generate a distinct distaste in the fastidious New Englander for the brash young first-generation Greek American. The killing point, the event which made James Bonar Auldfield a lifelong enemy of Athan Carras, came in the third year of med school, when Carras met and won Beth Cavendish.

She had the kind of face that instantly pulled a man's eyes, then pulled them back again for a second look. Not one of her features was perfect, yet somehow they combined to make her more than beautiful in the cover girl sense. She was, it didn't take long for Carras to realize, just *more*. And he discovered why: it was because behind those wonderfully combined features was an active intelligence that set Beth Cavendish apart. And the rest of her was everything it should have been.

She was the first woman Carras ever really fell for, the first to make him feel that there was a gap somewhere inside him and that she fitted into that gap exactly. There were at least a dozen men on the Yale campus who must have felt the same way about her, and one of them was the desperately shy James Bonar Auldfield. If there was ever a man designed to worship a woman from afar, it was he; and if there was ever a woman who could only be won by a man with a full flood of blood in his veins, it was Beth.

It was therefore the worst thing that could have happened to Auldfield that he heard noises late one night in the hallway outside his room. He got up out bed, wearing only boxer shorts, and opened the door to tell Carras—of course it would be Carras—to shut up and let decent people sleep. Instead, he found a tipsy Beth Cavendish, still warm and rosy from lovemaking, tiptoeing back to Carras's bed from the communal bathroom.

She was wearing one of Carras's shirts, unbuttoned, holding it together with one hand below her throat. When she saw Auldfield in the hallway, she giggled and raised an index finger to her lips. Unfortunately, she used the hand that had been holding the shirt closed, so that it fell open and revealed to the man of numbers an order of reality he had until then only guessed at.

Half asleep, Auldfield could do nothing but stare. And as he stared, the lower parts of his consciousness reacted as they were designed to do and sent a message to the contents of his boxer shorts, a message that was received and acted upon. She noticed—it was definitely noticeable—before he did, and her reaction turned the original giggle into a full sized embarrassed laugh.

She scampered quickly to Carras's door and went through it, leaving a horrified, devastated James Bonar Auldfield to step back into his room and close his own door, only to stand staring at its scarred and painted wood for a long moment—until he heard the sound of muffled laughter through the wall, and then clearly, in her voice, the words, "Bonar? His name is Bonar?" followed by something he didn't catch, and even more laughter.

He soon noticed that fellow students had taken to addressing him by his middle name and that they seemed to do so with a certain careful intonation or a definite twist to their lips. He never heard the nickname without hearing again the laughter of Carras and the woman for whom Auldfield secretly pined.

He never married, and on the day he heard that Beth Cavendish had finally left Athan Carras, taking their ten-year-old son Costas to California, he dined well at Mory's, the Yale dinner club, and had them bring up the crustiest bottle of port that its distinguished cellar held.

• • •

The Goldenberg operation was a resounding success. The edges of the multiple incisions cohered just as they had in the laboratory animals. Carras and Mason connected the patient's circulatory system to the new heart's left ventricle, then weaned the body off the bypass machine. The moment the new organ was given a jolt of electricity, it restarted and began to beat with a strong and steady rhythm. There were no shivers of fibrillation, and the patient did not even require any of the support medications that are routine in heart transplants.

Mason and Carras watched the monitors. Goldenberg's new, improved pump pushed blood through his resistant lungs like a victorious army routing an enemy from the battlefield. Cardiac output was optimum and the strong flow of oxygenated fluid cleansed the patient's other organs and tissues of the dangerous acids that had built up since his collapse. Cory Goldenberg would be leaving OR 15 a much healthier man. He was the first person in history to have a heart and a half—Carras's daring experimental operation.

Carras and Mason sutured and wired the layers of flesh and bone between the patient's heart and his skin, working swiftly and automatically. As Mason stitched up the outer incision, he said, "You know you're going to be famous, Ath. Or maybe I should say, even more famous."

"My old man used to tell me, 'Fame is just a stepping stone to destruction,'" Carras said, but he couldn't keep a smile from forming under his mask.

"Sure, yeah," Mason said, "'the paths of glory lead but to the grave,' and all that. But this path is going to lead to some goddamn gravy for Dr. Athan the Wonder Boy Carras."

Mason was right. Yale's publicity department was headed by a brisk young woman named Nancy Polwitz who had all the skills of a modern public relations professional and an assertiveness of personality that would have fit a Marine drill instructor. Informed that a Yale doctor had developed a revolutionary new procedure that had saved the life of a top Harvard cardiologist, Polwitz reacted like a one-woman air assault division.

"I need you to defer your caseload for the next week," she told Carras over the phone, the day after the operation. "I've booked a suite at the Park Plaza for two days of print interviews—*Time, Newsweek, People,* the usual dailies—then both *Dateline* and *20/20* want you in their New York studios. We're still talking to Oprah."

"Whoa," said Carras. "I can't walk away from my patients."

The publicity head's Midwestern twang became more pronounced when she encountered unreasonable people, which she defined as anybody who didn't agree with her. "Doctor," she said, "this is not about you. This is about the University. Yale has been very, very good to you. This is your chance to give a little back."

There were many other calls, including several from illustrious alumni and one from the President of the University. Carras caved in and called Nancy Polwitz and said she should go ahead and make arrangements.

She already had. "We're booked on the 8:15 Acela train to Manhattan tomorrow morning," she said. "I'll pick you up at 7:30. Don't pack any checked shirts or loud jackets. They tend to strobe on TV."

It was an exhilarating experience. Carras had heard movie stars complain about publicity tours with hour after hour of back-to-back interviews. And, true, it was exhausting to recount time after time how the dream had led to the idea, then how the procedure had been developed, and the life-or-death circumstances that had prompted its first application. But being treated like a celebrity, even only temporarily, felt good. He gave full credit to Craig Mason, but the reporters had dubbed the heart-and-a-half operation the Carras Procedure and the label stuck.

The medical reporter for *The New York Times* was the only one to ask the dark-side question. "What if it hadn't worked? What if Dr. Goldenberg had died?"

"I would have been devastated. He is my friend."

"Yet you risked his life with an untried procedure."

"It had been performed many, many times in the lab."

"On animals."

"The principles were the same," Carras said.

"But there were still unknown risks."

"Yes. Thank God all went well."

The reporter flipped a page in his notebook, read something written there, then said, "I understand you did not actually have the permission from the ethics committee to perform the procedure."

Carras was silent, wondering where the man had heard that. It was not in any background materials Nancy Polwitz had handed out. There could have been only one source.

"Doctor?" the reporter prodded.

Carras said, "The committee chair was unavailable. He was out in Montana without a phone or beeper."

"But you talked to someone from the committee." The reporter wasn't asking; he was looking for confirmation of something he already knew.

"Yes."

"Did you ask for permission to proceed?"

"Yes."

"But you did not receive it."

Carras chose his words carefully. "I was told it was my decision to make."

• • •

The coverage was almost unanimously positive—great new breakthrough, many lives to be saved—and the Harvard-Yale rivalry angle was featured prominently in most stories.

The *Times* write-up took a different tack, lauding the result but asking leading rhetorical questions about the "glaring absence of regulatory oversight for surgical experimentation." Nothing was said directly, but Carras felt the piece gave a distinct impression that he was some kind of scalpel-wielding maverick. The article ended in a series of open queries: "Will the success of the Carras Procedure encourage other surgeons to play God with their patients? And will the next high-risk experiment end in a life saved—or a life lost?"

Carras read the article in his office. After the second reading he threw the paper into the wastebasket and swore.

Charlie Vance had picked it up at the newsstand in the med center lobby and brought it over. He sat in the chair usually occupied by patients in for a pre-operative consultation. Vance said, "I looked up the reporter's cee-vee."

"Yeah?" Carras said, knowing there would be something to come.

"Harvard Med, Class of '82."

Carras made a confirmatory grunt deep in his throat.

Vance steepled his fingers, cocked his head to one side and raised his eyebrows. The resemblance to Nicholson was almost eerie. "Also, he prepped at Andover."

It took a moment to sink in. "Boner was at Andover," Carras said.

"Yep," his friend said then leaned back in his chair, his eyes roaming over the wall behind Carras, which was covered with certificates and diplomas, some framed letters from famous people whose hearts he had worked on, and slightly gaudy testimonial plaques from commercial agencies that polled

America's physicians and surgeons to find out who were the Best Doctors in America. "You know," Vance drawled, "if all that stuff ever pulls that wall down on you, we will have the best metaphor since Dr. Faustus for a man destroyed by his own success."

"Ha ha," said Carras and used his foot to push the Times deeper into the trash.

"I'll buy you dinner tonight," Vance said. "I'm not afraid that the fiery glow of your celebritude will consume me."

• • •

It was a good dinner and Carras came home to his empty apartment in a low-rise block on the campus still warmed by his friend's affection. In the hallway outside his door a man was leaning against the wall with an air of having waited some time. He was thirtyish in a well tailored, conservatively cut suit that could not compensate for a round-shouldered physique. His thin face was made to seem unnaturally elongated by a pointed chin and a well receded hairline, and the corners of his mouth had turned down so frequently that there were little creases there.

"Dr. Carras?" he said. "My name is Leonard Maigrot. I'd like to talk to you."

The man's hands were cold and his handshake perfunctory. Carras unlocked his door and said, "I'm not doing any more interviews."

"I'm not a reporter, doctor." He handed Carras his card. It showed nothing but his name and a phone number.

Carras needed to get to bed. He had to perform a transplant and repair an aortic aneurysm the next day, plus rounds and some teaching work. His friend Charlie Vance had once wondered if Carras needed sleep because he worked so hard, or if it was the other way round: maybe he worked too hard because fatigue would let him fall asleep the moment his head hit the pillow, and then he wouldn't have to lie there thinking about the things that hurt too much to think about.

"What do you want?" Carras asked Maigrot.

"It's a medical matter."

"Then make an appointment with my secretary. I don't see patients at my home." He stepped through the doorway, but Maigrot caught the edge of the door and did not let it close.

"I'm not a patient, and my employer would prefer to remain anonymous for the moment," he said.

"Let go of the door," Carras said.

Maigrot flinched a little at Carras's tone, but held his position. "I'd like to arrange for you to meet my employer. He'd like to make you an offer."

"What kind of offer?"

The man shrugged. "I don't know the details."

Carras had had enough. "Mr. Maigrot, I'm tired and I have to work tomorrow. Your employer can call my secretary or send me a letter or do whatever he likes, but you can tell him that I have a low tolerance for people who like to play games. Whatever he wants, if this is the way he intends to go about it, the answer is going to be no." He looked the man squarely in the eyes. "Now take your hand off the door."

Maigrot's long fingers lifted off the wood like the tendrils of a sea anenome moved by an idle current. "It would be a lot easier on everybody if you'd reconsider," he said. "I'll be in touch."

• • •

It was almost a month after the Goldenberg operation. Carras had completed his morning surgery and was in his office attending to a stack of correspondence, much of it generated by the publicity that Nancy Polwitz had orchestrated. The pioneering surgeon was in high demand for conferences and seminars.

Karen buzzed him on the intercom. "That reporter from the New York Times is on the line."

Carras grabbed for the phone. It was an opportunity to tell the snide insinuator what he thought of him, in detail. But the reporter didn't give him a chance. As soon as they were connected he said, "Dr. Carras, what is your reaction to the sudden death of Dr. Cory Goldenberg, apparently from complications of your untried surgical technique?"

• • •

Dr. Cory Goldenberg died in his sleep. At ten a.m., his assistant, concerned that her boss had missed two morning appointments and was not answering his phone or pager, called the police to check the home where the cardiologist had lived alone since the death of his wife. He was already in the first stages of rigor mortis.

The Times man had a beat on all the other major media—Carras was sure that was Auldfield's doing—and the scribe made a meal of it. He got little from Carras in the telephone ambush, just the surgeon's expression of shock and regret, but that was all he wanted. The shape of the piece was already in the reporter's head before he made the call.

Noted cardiologist Dr. Cory Goldenberg always warned against a too ready recourse to surgery for heart disease. Last month he went against his own teachings and put himself under the experimental knife of Dr. Athan Carras. Now he is dead.

What followed was more self-congratulation than reportage. The Times man reminded his readers that he alone had sounded a word of warning, cutting across the rest of the media's stream of adulation and gee-whiz celebrification of a self-willed doctor who may have gone well beyond the canon of medical ethics, lured by the *ignis fatui* of fame and professional acclaim.

The article wound its way toward an unsubtle allusion to Dr. Frankenstein, who unnaturally sewed dead parts together to create his own destruction, before concluding with a question: "Will the medical fraternity—especially those who wear a Yale alumni pin—close ranks around a rogue member, so that he may soon resume an apparently reckless course of human experimentation; or will they make of this case an unmistakable example that will save lives and restore public confidence in the profession and in the institution where this outrage was permitted to occur?"

The rest of the media pack followed the scent of blood. Although one or two voices mentioned that no cause of death had yet been established, the general tone of the coverage copied the Frankenstein motif. Some articles spun off into wide-eyed speculation on the possibility of harvesting organs from animals genetically altered to pass for human, at least at the DNA level. Others raised the prospect of mindless clones grown in tanks to provide organs, "like a junked parts-car out in the weeds, ready to supply a replacement set of whatever we need, on demand."

But whether the coverage stayed on the Goldenberg case or wandered out into the farthest frontiers of medicine, the role of Athan Carras remained central to the stories.

"You've become a symbol," Nancy Polwitz said. "Despite fifty years of doctor shows on TV, from Ben Casey to General Hospital to ER, half the country couldn't differentiate medical science from spells and potions. They have to rely on doctors as if they were an order of priests. When somebody comes along and says one of the priests is really doing black magic, a lot of people get scared."

She held up a supermarket tabloid with a cover photo of Carras. The flash of the photographer's strobe had caught him close up as he came out of his apartment block, making him look pale, and someone had retouched the image to enlarge his eyes, so that he looked slightly alien. The headline referred to him as Dr. Death.

"You're saying I'm a symbol of evil?" Carras said.

"Of fear," the PR woman said. "Until another one comes along, you're America's bogey man."

"But we don't even have the autopsy results. Cory was in his mid sixties. He might have died from a dozen unrelated causes."

"You'd better hope he did. In the meantime, no more interviews. This will die down."

"No fear of that," Carras said. "I don't even answer my home phone unless it first rings twice to let me know it's Karen."

• • •

The post-mortem examination of Dr. Cory Goldenberg showed that he died of cardiac tamponade, bleeding around the heart. He had bled from the pericardium, the sac that surrounds the heart and which is always irritated and inflamed after open heart surgery.

"It doesn't make any sense," Carras told Charlie Vance looking up from a print-out of the autopsy report that had been e-mailed to his office. "We solved that problem in the animal model. There's no way it should have happened."

"Let me see." Vance took the report and scanned the pages. "Did you have him on any blood thinners?" he said.

Carras shook his head. "No. He wanted to use an anti-coagulant because he was afraid clots might form at the anastomoses and he'd be at risk of stroke if they went to the brain. But it wasn't a problem in the animal trials and I talked him out of it. Why?"

"His blood was thinner than it should have been," Vance said, pointing to the notation on the autopsy report.

Carras reached for the phone. Two minutes later he was talking to Gulwar Singh, the pharmacist at Harvard Medical Center who had filled Cory Goldenberg's post-operative prescriptions. The pharmacist ran down a list of medications the cardiologist had been taking, immunosuppressive drugs, diuretics and some blood pressure pills, then he said a word that made Carras sit up.

"Did you say Coumadin?" Carras said.

"Yes, Coumadin," the pharmacist said. "Five milligrams daily." It was a strong dose of a powerful blood thinner.

Carras thanked him and hung up. "Well, that's it," he told Vance. "He must have still been worried about clotting and decided to prescribe for himself. The blood thinner caused bleeding from the pericardium and that caused Cory's death. I'm in the clear."

"Don't count on it," Vance said.

"They can't blame me if he didn't do what I prescribed."

"Don't count on it," Vance repeated.

"In any court of law..." Carras began.

"This ain't no court of law," Vance said, dropping into his Nicholson drawl. "It's the court of public opinion. Case closed."

• • •

There was no change in the tone of the coverage. The details of the autopsy results were reported but the story now had its own momentum. Many Americans were scared by their own thoughts about where medical science was taking them, and Athan Carras had become the focus of their fear.

"It will die down," Nancy Polwitz had said. But it wasn't dying down. The media maintained that the public was "looking for closure." The PR woman translated that phrase as the media's way of saying they wanted a head to roll—and they knew whose head they wanted.

Yale's Board of Governors convened a special panel and summoned Athan Carras to appear before it.

"Should I get a lawyer?" Carras asked Vance. He knew the ethicist was closer to the powers that were than he had ever been. Many of them had gone to the same schools.

"Only if you want to make things worse," his friend told him. He let his eyes wander over Carras's collection of plaques and testimonials then out toward the morgue. "What I'm hearing is, this isn't about you any more. It's about the University. Some important alumni are phoning. There's many a quiet word over a drink."

"I didn't do anything wrong," Carras said.

"This country occasionally executes people who can say the same thing," Vance said. "What counts is not whether you did anything wrong, but whether they can make a case against you."

"And can they?"

Vance stuck out his lower lip and spread his hands. "Boner has been a busy little beaver. Everybody has heard from him, quietly, and he's saying he did not give you the HIC's permission to operate on Cory."

"He said it was up to me."

Vance made a face that looked like he'd just tasted acid. "Then they've got you."

"That's not fair."

"Fair has got nothing to do with it. You bound yourself to do what the committee said. The committee said wait. You didn't wait. Ethically, you're in breach."

"But Cory would have died," Carras said.

"Cory did die."

"But that wasn't my..."

"Doesn't matter."

Carras said, "I need a lawyer."

He reached for the phone on his desk, but Vance put out his hand and stopped him. "No."

"Tell me, Charlie," Carras said. "Whose side are you on in this, mine or the University's?"

"As it happens," Vance said, "I'm on both sides."

"Good trick," said Carras. "Want to tell me how it's done?"

"You're a problem for the University. You haven't done anything wrong, but you have got the press all atwitter. If Yale does nothing about you, the fuss will continue. Some alumni checks will be smaller—maybe they won't get written at all. So something has got to be done about you."

"When do you come over to my side?"

"Now," said Vance. "You're in a position to help the University by making this thing go away."

"By resigning? Give up tenure?" Carras kept his voice level, but he was aware of a creeping sensation around the edges of his mind. His work was his life. He had given up so much to be who and what he was; the thought of losing it all brought a chill. His face felt suddenly cold, as if all the blood had drained from it.

His friend saw Carras grow pale and hurried to reassure him. "No, no, no. Nothing so drastic. You admit to the technical breach of ethics. You accept a mild censure—maybe a temporary suspension of your operating privileges—and do a little research for a while. The media have their pound of flesh. It all blows over and you go back to normal."

"How long a suspension?"

"Few weeks. Six at the most."

Carras looked at his friend. "Charlie," he said, "while I'm sitting here am I hearing just your personal opinion or am I now in a negotiation with Yale?"

"Depends on whether you find the scenario acceptable or not."

"If I do, it's an offer, isn't it, Charlie? But what if I don't find it acceptable? Then what?"

Vance thought about it for a moment, then said, "Some doors it's better not to open. Ath, this is a blip in a long and brilliant career."

It was Carras's turn to do some thinking. "What kind of research? I've done everything I can do with the heart-and-a-half."

"Before you got into that project, weren't you doing something with cold water?" Vance said.

The question stopped Carras. He hadn't thought of the other project in months. Before the heart-and-a-half research had begun he had conducted some very limited and preliminary investigations of a phenomenon called deep hypothermic circulatory arrest. DHCA was the rapid chilling of a patient's body by cooling the blood as it passed through a heart-lung machine. Then, unlike conventional open heart surgery, the heart-lung machine was turned off. The patient had no pulse, no blood pressure, no EKG or EEG activity—nothing. It was a state scarcely distinguishable from death.

The way the phenomenon worked was only partly understood, but the result was clear: animals put into DHCA entered a state that could only be called suspended animation; their condition did not deteriorate and when revived, after several hours, they came back as if the intervening time hadn't happened.

The technique was already being used in human patients for complex aortic surgery that required an operating field entirely free of blood flow. For

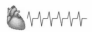

periods of up the three-quarters of an hour, the technique had been proved to be safe. Rarely had there been an incidence of a patient suffering adverse effects from the procedure.

DHCA's potential implications for organ transplants were immense. Instead of carrying harvested organs from one city to another, depriving them of oxygen and nutrients so that they inevitably deteriorated en route, donors might be kept "on ice" and transported to where their organs were needed.

Even more promising, patients who were hard to match could be cooled into a virtual state of suspended animation while they waited for a suitable organ to appear. Ultimately, DHCA might offer what cryogenic freezing never could: the potential to suspend a living patient with an incurable disease until, possibly years later, a cure was found.

Carras had "borrowed" a heart-lung machine and set up in an unused corner of a lab to conduct two small-scale experiments: he had kept a guinea pig and a rabbit "suspended" for three days before reviving them unharmed. But then the heart-and-a-half project had shown promise and he had put suspended animation on the shelf and almost forgotten about it.

"What are you saying, Charlie?" he asked his friend. "If I take one for the team, the way will be smoothed toward a substantial grant for DHCA research?"

His friend tented his fingers over his small pot belly and leaned back in Carras's visitor's chair. "That's exactly what I'm saying, Ath."

"And if I stand up for myself? Get a lawyer?"

"Oh, you'd probably win in court."

"I hear a 'but' coming."

"But you'd lose everywhere else."

Carras said nothing, thinking about it. It went against the grain to admit fault when he had done nothing wrong.

Vance said, "Don't make too much of it, Ath. It's just one of those little curve balls that life sometimes throws us. Worst thing to do is to swing at it as hard as you can."

"Maybe you're right," Carras said. "Who was it who said, 'Surgery is simple; it's life that's complicated?'"

"Actually, I think that was me," Vance said.

• • •

When the coverage had begun to build, Carras changed his home number to an unlisted one. So he was surprised when it rang the evening after his conversation with Charlie Vance and the voice on the other end belonged to Leonard Maigrot.

"My employer is still very interested in meeting you."

"How did you get this number?" Carras said.

"We would send a jet."

"I'm not interested," Carras said.

"I think you will be."

"No."

"He won't accept no for an answer, not without your hearing his offer. You would be well advised to meet with him."

"Is that a threat?" Carras said.

"I'm not authorized to make threats, Dr. Carras. Let's say it's a suggestion."

Carras's patience was wearing thin. "If you bother me again, I'll call the police."

Maigrot laughed. "That would be going a bit too far," he said. "I can assure you that you'll be interested in the offer."

"Leave me alone."

"My employer says otherwise, doctor," Maigrot said. "We'll be in touch again soon."

Chapter 3

When he was in the OR, Athan Carras could reduce his entire world to a space no larger than a foot wide and two feet long. A former classmate, now a psychiatrist who treated famous athletes who had temporarily misplaced the ability to hit or throw a ball, had once observed Carras at the operating table. He remarked that he had never seen such intensity of focus, not even in a major-league superstar.

Carras had invited the man to consider the alternative. "Do you want my mind wandering through my personal life while your heart is beating under my hand?"

This morning, in OR-15 of the Yale Medical Center, Carras had forced the Goldenberg mess from his mind. His world was bounded by the two square feet of flesh that were the mediastinum—the region between the left and right lungs—of a ten-year-old boy named Jordan Farina.

The child was already a veteran of cardiac surgery. He had come into the world like a jigsaw puzzle with a piece gone. If the missing part had been a little toe or the genetically determined muscle that allows some people to roll the tongue into a tube, the lack wouldn't have made much difference. But Jordan was missing a piece of his heart.

Like any other mammal, Jordan Farina should have had a four-chambered heart, containing a left and a right ventricle and a left and a right atrium, a four-part pump fashioned from an incredibly durable and uncomplaining muscle. But baby Jordan's left ventricle, the part that pumps blood from the body, was just not there. And three chambers—though it is a number that works for reptiles—could not keep the infant alive for long.

He first went under the knife at four days old. The procedure, for all its sophistication of technique, was what a mechanic would have called a running repair. It was enough to keep the child alive until, at four months, the pediatric cardio team could open him up again and perform the second phase of the process.

Like home renovators rescuing an old house, the doctors rearranged the three remaining chambers of Jordan's heart, removing dividers and creating connections to establish a new floor plan. A year later, the surgeons reconvened over the child's open chest a third time, and completed the transformation of his ill-made heart. When they sewed him up, they had rebuilt the organ so that it would function with only two chambers, a design that works well enough for fish and tadpoles. It should have let Jordan Farina grow up to lead a relatively normal life.

But something went wrong, shortly after the boy's tenth birthday. The renovations were not holding. No more repairs and realignments could be made. It would have to be a new heart. He was admitted to the Coronary Care Unit at YMC and placed on the artificial heart known as a left ventricular assist device. The LVAD, a machine the size of a coconut, would pump the child's blood for him while he waited to see if a matching donor could be found.

Five days after the LVAD began to clank inside Jordan's chest—two days after Cory Goldenberg died in his sleep—a thirteen-year-old girl hanged herself in her room at a well regarded prep school. She had been bullied past the limits of despair by a clique of monsters in fashionable color coordinates. After their daughter was pronounced brain dead in the emergency room, the weeping parents were approached by Angela De Laura, a motherly nurse with eyes that said she was acquainted with sorrow. She was Yale's transplant coordinator.

She had already checked the dying girl's blood type against Jordan's. They matched. If the cross-match of donor blood cells with Jordan's blood was also good, there was a fair chance the poor girl's heart would live on to beat in they boy's chest.

De Laura spoke the words that, though she had so often said them before, had never become easy, never routine. The dead girl's mother must have been gardening when the police came to tell her. She was in jeans and a sweatshirt, the knees a little damp with soil. Now she stared at De Laura without comprehension, as if she had been spoken to in Urdu or Swahili. Then the woman's face was suddenly distorted by a spasm that seemed to shoot down through the rest of her like an electrical charge, twisting her torso and crooking her limbs at harsh, ungainly angles. As quickly as it had come, it was past. It was as if all the rigidity had gone out of her bones. She turned and buried her face in the angle where her husband's neck met his chest, and her body heaved with the first of the sobs.

The father was an open-faced man with crinkles at the corners of his eyes. The little lines deepened now as he looked at De Laura over his wife's hair that shivered from the spasms wracking her body and said, "Let some good come of this. Some good for somebody. Go and do it."

They took a lymph node from the comatose girl and placed it in a laboratory dish with some of the boy's serum, the watery part of his blood that contained the antibodies that would react if his body was likely to reject the donor's tissue. It was like a transplant in a test tube, a mimic in miniature of the procedure itself. The lab tech phoned De Laura two hours after the cells were harvested. "You've got a green light," he said.

• • •

Carras had already placed the so-called purse-string stitches on the boy's major arteries and veins in preparation for the tubes of the heart-lung machine that would take over the business of providing blood and oxygen to the body's tissues. Now he swiftly opened the blood vessels and inserted the garden hose-sized tubings into them, drawing the stitches tight so that the arteries and veins closed snugly around the tubes.

"Take it away, Dino," he said to the man squatting on the kindergarten-sized stool below the operating table. Dr. Martin Denobis, the talented perfusionist Carras preferred to work with, did not look away from the readouts on the heart-lung machine, a low-slung device that despite thirty years of development and refinement still resembled something from a Rube Goldberg cartoon. "Check," he said.

"Okay," said Carras, "let's get this misshapen thing out of the kid and give him one that works." His scalpel moved quickly and with perfect precision to separate the organ from the boy it had failed. It was a moment that always gave Carras a visceral gratification.

As he lifted the lump of lifeless tissue clear of the boy's narrow chest, the scrub nurse raised a stainless-steel bucket. The defective heart flopped onto the bottom of the container with a dull, wet sound.

Yale was a teaching hospital, and for many operations Carras was assisted by a surgical resident, a recently graduated general surgeon who was learning the specialized art of rebuilding hearts. But the Farina operation was one of those cases where he preferred to have calm, well centered Lynnette Feldsher as his first assistant. Her small, fine boned hands were delicate but they would unerringly hold the coronary arteries perfectly still while Carras sewed. He had worked with too many residents who hadn't yet learned that absolute control of every motion was essential in a surgeon's hands.

Equally important, Carras believed, was absolute control of every emotion in the surgeon's own heart. He had told the interviewer from *People* magazine that when he was operating, he thought of himself as an ice man: no sentiment, no feelings, just the cold purity of skill and concentration. He hadn't meant to let that thought slip through his guard, but in her own way, the interviewer had been almost as good at opening people up as Carras himself.

But he had kept the whole truth from her; beneath the ice man was another Athan Carras, a man who was possessed by a fierce joy that blazed up when his hands cut and joined and sewed to make people whole again. As Chief of Cardiothoracic Surgery at Yale, he was well recompensed for his work; but at moments like this, when Lynnette brought him the deep basin of cold, sterile water that held the donor heart, the heart that Carras would use to restore life to the supremely vulnerable child whose chest lay open before him, those were the times when he believed he would have happily done it for minimum wage. It was as close as a man ever got to playing God.

There was another level beneath the joy, but it was a place he went to only in dreams or in those rare and fleeting moments when some tiny signal—the way a woman's hair shone in the sunlight, or a child's shout from a playground—would call up a memory of the time before he had let himself become the ice man. He had pushed the memories down and away, but they were still there somewhere.

Together, he and Lynnette inspected the donor heart. The organ's buoyancy made it float up to the surface and they kept pushing it down so that it would remain cool as they inspected and prepared it for implantation. Although the heart had been examined immediately after being harvested from the donor, Carras made a final, detailed inspection now. A surgeon believes first what his own fingers and eyes tell him, he would always tell his students; any test can be wrong, any result involves a margin of error.

Now Carras looked inside the chambers to rule out any congenital flaws. He checked the arteries: it was unlikely that there would be any hardening in a thirteen-year-old donor, but among heart transplant surgeons, perfectionism is not considered a character fault. He hadn't minded telling that to the *People* interviewer.

The heart was good. Carras and Lynnette quickly trimmed and shaped the four major structures that led out of the organ so that they would connect to the corresponding arteries and veins of Jordan Farina. Then Carras gently lifted the heart from its basin and placed it on a sponge soaked in cold fluid that Lynnette positioned to the left of the incision in the boy's chest. She softly rested her left hand on the heart while her right went into the boy's chest to hold the first chamber for Carras to sew.

He put three large stitches into the first two chambers to be connected, extending the sterile thread to the appropriate connective structure on the donor heart and the recipient's chest. When the stitches were in place, Lynnette positioned the organ over the hole in Jordan's chest so that the threads descended into the incision like the cords of a parachute. Then Carras gently put strain on the threads as Lynnette delicately lowered the heart into place.

Now the rest was automatic. Lynnette would hold each chamber in turn and Carras would finely stitch the connections, beginning with the left atrium at the top of the heart, which sat deeper in the body than the other three structures and would be unreachable once the organ was fully in place. Next came the right atrium, the heart's intake structure which accepts blood from the body. Then they connected the aorta of the heart to Jordan's own aorta, creating the unified high-pressure vessel that would carry blood to the body, pumped by the strength of the donor organ's strong left ventricle.

As he placed the last stitch in the aorta, Carras said, "Five hundred milligrams of Solumedrol IV now." Paul Lefebre, the anesthesiologist, reflexively repeated the words to confirm that the medication was being administered. Lefebre was a dependable specialist; it was unlikely that he would forget to infuse the powerful steroid without which any new heart would be swiftly rejected by a recipient's body. But every heart transplant surgeon in the world said precisely those words at this stage of the procedure, before blood flow to the new heart was re-established.

Carras had said the words automatically and automatically registered the anesthesiologists' response. But now, for the first time in an operating theater, something was interfering with his concentration, something that niggled at the back of his mind like a tiny, unfocused itch.

He shook his head, only a twitch, and this time he was sure he noticed a reaction in Lynnette, a slight widening of her calm gray eyes. Carras cleared his throat and willed himself to concentrate on the work in front of him. The boy deserved no less than one hundred percent of what the surgeon brought to the table.

The boy deserves... He actually heard the words in his head, in that anonymous voice with which he verbalized his own thoughts. *The boy deserves a heart.* And then he heard an echo of another voice, Beth's voice, saying, *He's your son and he deserves a father.*

Now Carras realized what was happening. It was because the patient was a boy, and a ten-year-old boy at that—the same age as Costas had been the last time Carras had seen him. And because yesterday his ex-wife had called, the first time in a long time that they had talked. She'd seen the coverage that had made him America's bogey man and had called to wish him well. Then they had talked about their son.

Carras consciously focused his mind back to the work under his hands. The crucial moment in every transplant operation was fast approaching: the point when the implanted heart must be made to beat again in its new home as it had beaten in the donor's body. The new heart was always at its weakest in the crucial minutes after it was restarted. Even though it had been kept cool, which induced a kind of suspended animation in the resilient cardiac muscle of which it was made, its tissues had been deprived of oxygen since it had been separated from the brain-dead donor's circulatory system.

As he set the last few stitches, Carras's sensitive fingers and experienced eyes noted the heart's continuing fibrillation, an erratic and ineffectual quivering that said the organ was alive but not yet functioning. As he completed the last suture, he felt the heart's continued trembling in the boy's chest.

Moment of truth, he told himself, but to Paul Lefebre he said, with the ice man's calm, "Lidocaine, 150 milligrams, please."

The lidocaine was a powerful antiarrhythmic drug, designed to restore a fibrillating heart to a normal rhythm. It ought to act immediately. But as the surgical team stared into the cavity of Jordan Farina's mediastinum, the boy's heart—definitely his now, not the dead girl's any longer—produced no more than tiny tremors.

Come on, said the voice in Athan Carras's head. *The boy deserves...* but he cut that thought off with a surgeon's decisiveness and said aloud, "Let's have the paddles. Ten joules."

They were like two large fly swatters. Carras positioned them on either side of the heart, and nodded to the nurse. He could tell from the way her surgical mask moved that she was biting her lip as she pressed the red button on the defibrillator. The machine made a sound like a basement furnace kicking in on a cold night and shot its charge through Jordan's heart. The boy's frail body arched like a blue rainbow under the sterile drapes. Carras withdrew the paddles and placed his right index finger on the organ's surface, but felt only a tiny shiver.

Come on, boy, he thought. *You want to live. Come on.* Without turning his head, he said, "Dino, let's...," and he was about to tell the perfusionist to increase the pressure of the blood flowing into the heart, to red-line the heart-lung machine at its maximum flow of eight liters per minute and enrich the organ's tissues with life-giving oxygen, making it safe and appropriate to try the electric shock again. But as the words were on his lips, he felt the shiver under his finger become a shudder, a strong one.

The dead girl's heart convulsed in the living boy. It clenched and released, like a fist closing its grip then loosening. There was a pause, which lasted a long moment, then the heart beat again, then once more, and now it began to pulse with a good rhythm. The surgical team watched and under their masks there were smiles. It didn't matter how many times you did this, Carras knew, the moment when a new heart began to beat was like nothing else. "Houston," he said, "we have lift-off."

In fact, with the heart-lung machine still doing the organ's work for it, while supplying fresh, oxygen-rich blood, the load-free heart was growing stronger with each regular beat, almost jumping out of the boy's chest. "Wean us off bypass," Carras said to the perfusionist, and watched as the new organ took up the strain it was evolved to bear.

It was fine. Carras removed the heart-lung tubing and closed the layers of the boy's open chest, stitching flesh and wiring bone as he had done so many times before. It was a routine activity, one he probably could have done in his sleep, but it carried with it a warm sense of completion, like the last extended chord of a romantic symphony.

"Good job, team," he said. "As always." But as he said the familiar words, he felt again the sensation of something tugging at the edge of his mind, like a toddler's hand pulling at the hem of a parent's coat. Well, he knew it had to be faced, and so he turned his thoughts toward the matter he had been so careful to suppress while he had been the ice man focused on Jordan Farina's heart.

It was time he reconnected with his son, now nineteen and finishing his first year in computer science at Stanford. It was not going to be easy. Carras had a hard time dealing with strong, raw emotion, had made a practice of not dealing with it. He tended to stiffen up and talk in short, clipped phrases.

But he had promised Beth he would do it. She was right: the boy deserved a father. But it wouldn't have been easy even if Carras had been good at this kind of thing. Costas had refused all contact with his father since he had got into the cab that took him and Beth to the airport, nine years before, and had sent back birthday cards and Christmas presents unopened.

• • •

The extraordinary committee on ethics and practices met in a seminar room on the ground floor of a building that had been ivy-covered when Lee surrendered at Appomattox. It was a wet March morning, with the tail end of an Atlantic winter storm throwing itself at the mullioned windows. The somberness of the sky seemed to leach into the room and darken even the electric lights.

The media had not been allowed into the proceedings, but a news release had been prepared in advance. Nancy Polwitz had shown the final draft to Carras, and he had approved its dignified wording. Yale's Provost presided over the brief proceedings which took place around a walnut table at which George Washington was said to have dined. A distinguished scholar in his own right, the old man said only a few words, to which Carras made an even briefer reply. The proctor said a few more words and it was done.

Charlie Vance sat through the business with Carras and put his arm around his friend's shoulders when it was over. James Bonar Auldfield had been summoned in case there was any need for him to speak. There was none, but he smiled a quiet smile as he left the room.

Carras went back to his office. "It isn't fair," Karen said when she saw him. She wiped at one eye.

Carras put his arm around her the way Vance had done with him. "No," he said, "not fair. But at least it's over."

He had been relieved of teaching duties during the term of his suspension. For the first time since he was a freshman, he was on campus with nothing in particular to do.

Karen put her head through the doorway. "Beth called," she said.

Carras thanked her and reached for the phone. It was time to speak to his son.

• • •

There had been a marriage, and Carras had been a part of it. But not enough of a part of it, obviously, because the marriage had dwindled and died, and he couldn't say truthfully to himself that he hadn't let it happen. There had been a child too, a strong-minded, curly-haired boy he and Beth had named Costas, after Athan's grandfather.

The old man used to say that the child was the living image of what Athan had been when he was a loud but miniature whirlwind racing around the little clapboard house in the less than fashionable Philadelphia neighborhood where he had grown up, or getting underfoot at the service station on Market Street, where the older Costas had gone to work as a mechanic after immigrating from Greece, and which he ended up owning.

Judging by the snapshots that Beth sent faithfully from California two or three times a year, nineteen-year-old Costas could have been plucked from one of the old photos that owned the wall above the mantelpiece in his grandfather's house—all those bygone Carrases, stiff and serious in black suits with collarless white shirts buttoned up to the top, thick mustaches tapering out to points like the horns of ancient bulls. Snip the image of the boy from the bright background of sun-warmed stucco and jacaranda blossoms on Beth's back porch, decolorize the image and paste him in among the old-time Carrases, those fishermen from Crete, and Costas would have fit. He had the same jutting jaw, the same dark eyes under uncompromising brows, the same short vertical crease between those brows, the line that says, this is a serious man.

Athan Carras wondered if his son smiled much, the way people were supposed to, out there in California. He never did it in the photos, but always stared into the lens of Beth's camera with a face that challenged the eyes that would regard his image. Perhaps, Carras thought, he only reserved that look for pictures that his mother would be sending to his father, the width of a continent away. Perhaps the boy smiled and let some light into his eyes the rest of the time. Carras hoped so.

The divorce had been more sad than bitter, reflecting a marriage that hadn't cracked apart but had just faded away. Carras moved to an apartment on campus, the same one he lived in now, while Beth and Costas stayed in the nice old house on Ronan Street that they had bought in the second year of their marriage, when the child was on the way. There was a court-ordered schedule for twice-weekly visits, but they hadn't gone well from the start.

Carras and Beth consulted a counselor, a carefully spoken woman who wore clothes that matched the beige color scheme of her office. She said that the boy blamed his father for abandoning him—those were her words; Costas had told her, "He doesn't care about us"—and that it might be some time before he got over the initial resentment. When Carras came to see his son, the boy refused to leave his bedroom, and would only shout through the locked door, "Go away."

Carras and Beth decided that there was no sense in trying to press the child while he was in pain. Let things settle down and he would come around. But months passed and Costas didn't come around. "He's a Carras," the boy's grandmother said. "The world changes. They don't. They don't know how."

A year after the final decree, fourteen months after Athan Carras had last stood outside Costas's locked door, Beth and the boy went west to take over a vineyard and winery that an affectionate uncle had left her. She had always had a feel for wine and—growing up in a family that would have had "Sir" and "Lady" attached to their names if it had not been for the disagreements of 1776—she had been able to develop as sophisticated a palate as any on the northeastern seaboard.

"Sometimes a great distance can have the same effect on the mind as a long time," she told her former husband. "After he's been out there a few months or a year, all this may seem less painful than it does now. Just give him time."

Athan Carras had agreed. He might have fought the planned move in the courts, could have demanded at least alternate shared custody, the boy shuttling back and forth from coast to coast, a few months here, a few months there. But that would have been hard on Costas. And though he never said it to anyone, not even to himself, Carras knew that it would be easier on him to make a clean break, to put it all behind him and concentrate on doing what he did best, in the aseptic sterility of OR 15, where the cuts were straight and precise and the wounds could be stitched closed and trusted to heal.

He agreed with his departing ex-wife. Better to let the distance intervene and wait for the boy to get over the pain. But the boy never did get over it, and now it had been nine years. It came as a shock to Athan Carras that so much time had gone by. He had always meant to make an effort, yet somehow things had got in the way. Now the boy was a man who didn't know his father, and all the father knew of the boy was a memory. Beth was right, it was no way for things to be. A boy deserves a father, and a father owes it to his son to offer himself.

• • •

When she had first called after Cory Goldenberg's death, Beth had suggested a way for Carras and his son to reconnect.

"Do you still have the Pantera?" she asked.

"You bet," Carras said. She was talking about his 1986 De Tomaso Pantera, the GTS model with a tweaked engine and suspension that was Athan Carras's only passion outside of medicine.

Though designed and built by the visionary Tom Tjaarda at Italy's famous Ghia coachworks, the sports car was powered by a honking great Australian Ford vee-eight shipped over from Detroit. The big engine was positioned midline, so it throbbed like a gloating giant right behind the driver's seat.

The car was the only thing in Carras's life, besides Beth Cavendish, that he ever just had to have. He saw one in a Lincoln-Mercury dealer's window in New Haven when he was still an intern at Yale. It was fly yellow and he couldn't believe the lines of the thing. He went home and told Beth that when he started to make decent money, a Pantera was the first thing he was going to buy. And it was.

Beth had encouraged him. "It's good to see you excited about something besides work," she had said. "God, Ath, you need to loosen up a little."

But there had been nothing loose about Athan Carras when he was behind the wheel of the Pantera. He had driven the high-performance car with the same intensity of focus that he brought to the operating theater. But when Costas was old enough, he had sometimes strapped the boy into the passenger seat. His son had loved the surge of acceleration.

Beth's voice came down the phone line from California. "I have a cunning plan," she said. It sounded like a catch phrase Carras was supposed to recognize, from TV or a movie, but he didn't.

"Tell me," he said.

"Costas was at the mall with his friends a few weeks ago. They saw a Pantera. It just about blew him away."

"Must be in the genes," Carras said. He always forgot how much he liked hearing her voice. "He didn't remember? I used to take him out in it when he was little."

"No." There was a pause as if she was looking for the right words. "He doesn't remember much since we came out here. Grandpa and Grandma, he knows them and the old house on Market Street. But our life back then, there's almost nothing. It's as if he wiped it all away, made himself forget."

"Oh, Jesus," Carras said. He didn't know what to say. A silence grew as he sought for the right words, but they all seemed to have hidden themselves.

Beth broke the tension. "Yeah, well," she said. "So I let him go on about the Pantera for a while, then I mentioned you used to have one."

"And?"

"And now I'm going to mention that you still have one."

"Ah," Carras said. "It is a cunning plan." He tried to put a smile in his voice.

She heard the tone and echoed it. "Well, I'm sure you weren't just attracted by my radiant beauty."

The conversation had taken a strange bounce, Carras thought. "Certainly not," he said, "I thought your brain was quite beautiful, too. I particularly liked the curve of your medulla oblongata."

"Why Dr. Carras, the things you say." She paused, and as the silence lengthened he wondered if she was feeling as odd about the tone of the conversation as he was.

"Beth," he began, but but and then nothing came but the emotions. He tried for words again, "I wish..."

He heard her sigh and knew the moment was over. "Let's just talk about Costas," she said. Her voice was brisk and upbeat now. "I was thinking I could suggest that you might arrange for Costas to get behind the wheel of that Pantera, maybe take a trip down the old Pacific Coast Highway."

"I see," he said.

"I mean the two of you," she said. "A little get-reacquainted trip."

"I get you." Now it was his turn to pause.

"So what do you think?" she said.

"We haven't talked in so long."

"I know, but..." she said, and left it hanging.

The boy deserves a father. I owe it to him. Carras had spent a lifetime controlling life-or-death situations; he ought to be able to handle a phone conversation. "Okay," he said. "If Costas wants to do it, I'm in. I'll call him."

• • •

Nancy Polwitz had been right: Carras's suspension was on front pages and near the top of newscasts for a day. There were a few editorials, then it was over. The pack moved on to the next scent of blood. Carras waited a couple more days then phoned his son. Beth answered and they talked briefly.

"I wanted to wait until I wasn't America's bogey man," he said. "I didn't know how Costas would feel about it."

"Don't worry," she said. "If anything, it makes you more interesting. Remember, it was your medical career that was the problem. Seeing you take it in the shorts ought to make Costas lean a little more in the direction of forgiving you."

"Forgiving me?" he said.

"Well, isn't that what we're working toward?" Beth said.

He'd never actually said the word to himself and hearing it now from his former wife jolted him. But she was right. It wasn't just about "reconnecting" or "getting back together" with his son. Costas had not just been "emotional" or subject to some childish fit of pique. He had been hurt and Carras had been responsible for the pain.

The past couple of weeks had taught Carras something about undeserved suffering. "You're right," he said. "It is about forgiveness."

"He's in his room," Beth said. "I'll try to get him to take the phone."

He heard her footsteps on a hard surface, not fading as if she were walking away from the phone but remaining loud. She must be carrying a portable through the house, he realized, and wondered what the house was like, then what she was like in that house that he had never seen except in the backgrounds of photographs. He heard her voice calling Costas's name, as if through a closed door, and a muffled rumble of a reply. *Deep voice*, he thought. *A Carras.*

Then the sound was cut off and he knew that Beth had put her hand over the phone's mike so that he would not hear the argument as his son declined to talk to him and the boy's mother fought on for both of them. Another silence stretched itself out until Carras wondered if some computer program at the phone company, recognizing that no signal had moved on the line for the prescribed number of minutes, had cut the connection.

Then he heard a rustle and a throat clearing, and the deep voice said a gruff, "Hello."

"Costas," Carras said and froze, because what was he supposed to say? This is your father? The boy knew who he was talking to. Please forgive me? Too blunt and too early, guaranteed to elicit a "no" that would later be hard for his son to climb down from, even though the true answer might be "not yet."

But he couldn't say nothing, so Carras cleared his throat, hearing it sound just the same as when Costas had done it, and said, "How are you?"

"I'm okay."

"Your mom says you're doing well in school."

"Yeah."

"Well, good."

"Yeah."

Carras heard Beth saying something in the background, then Costas's voice, away from the phone, saying, "What do you want from me?"

Beth's voice again: just the tone, not the words, then Costas back on the line with, "Mom says you want to ask me something."

Carras took a breath. "Yeah," he said. "She said you liked a Pantera you saw out there."

"It was all right." He was not giving anything away.

"She tell you I still have the Pantera?"

"Yeah."

"Well, I was thinking about bringing it out there, take a vacation. Road trip."

"Uh huh," Costas said.

There was a world of caution in those two syllables, Carras thought. "I was wondering if you'd like to try her out, maybe take her down the coast highway."

A silence, then, "I dunno."

"Doesn't have to be any big deal. Just drive and see the country."

"Yeah, well, maybe."

"When are you free?"

"I dunno. Got a lot of stuff to do. Stanford's pretty demanding."

"Yeah," said Carras. "I hear you got a major scholarship."

"I did all right," his son said.

"You sure did."

There was a silence then. Carras was unsure of where to take the conversation. He didn't want to push. The worst thing, he knew, would be to come on as the big decision-maker, pushing to set a date for the trip. Probably things had gone as far as they were going to go today. He said, "I'll let you know when I'm likely to be coming out, okay?"

"Yeah, okay."

"I guess I'd better talk to your mom again."

"All right. She's right here."

Carras didn't want to let him go. "Hey, Costas?"

"I'm still here."

Carras wanted to say something about what he was feeling, some words that would make a connection, but he was long out of practice. An inner voice was warning him off. *Don't go blurting out some feel-good psychobabble.* Instead, he said, "Good to talk to you." In his head, he added the word, *son.*

There was a pause, then, "Yeah, me too. Here's mom."

He heard the sound of a door closing, then the footsteps on the hard floor and Beth's voice came, quiet, "I'm thinking that went well."

Carras felt the way he had after his first time at a podium, delivering a presentation to a medical conference—a feeling of deliverance coupled with a sense of grateful wonder that he had somehow got through it without choking on his own tongue. To Beth he said, "Yes, it was good. It was a beginning."

"I'm glad. He'll start getting tied up with exams pretty soon, but by the end of April he'll be free and clear. Can you set aside some time in early May?"

"No problem. My time is pretty much my own for the foreseeable future."

"God, Ath, I'm sorry," she said. "I know how much your work means to you. Hell, I ought to."

"I'm sorry," he said. "About all of it."

"It took me a while to realize you couldn't really help it," she said. "Opening people up and fixing them is not just what you do. It's who you are."

"That's very understanding, considering that it was me being who I am that busted up our marriage."

He heard a soft laugh, then she said, "Well, I wasn't all that understanding nine years ago. Guess I'm like wine—give me a few years and I mellow."

He couldn't think of anything to say. No, he corrected himself, he could think of plenty of things he might say at this moment but he didn't know if any single one of them was the right thing to say.

"Well, nobody said life was supposed to be easy," Beth said. "We've come out okay. We get you two back together, it can be all right."

She asked him what he was going to do and he told her about the suspended animation research. "That's sounds interesting," she said.

"Yeah, it may be."

"Sure. You'll discover something like you always do and save a whole new bunch of people."

She made him laugh. It was the first time he had laughed in more days than he could remember. He said he would call her when he knew what his schedule would be and they said goodbye. After he hung up, he sat at his desk for a while, not doing anything, just thinking about Beth and the boy. For the first time in a long time, it felt good to think about them.

Karen buzzed him. "The Chairman of the Space Committee called. They've set aside some space for you in the Boyer Building. And there's a budget allocation for supplies and equipment."

"That was fast," he said.

"It's the least they can do, after what they..."

He cut her off, "It's okay, Karen. They didn't burn me at the stake."

She harrumphed. He'd never heard a woman make the noise, but that was the only word for it.

"I'll go over and look at the space," he said. "Then I guess I'll go home. I've got dinner with Charlie tonight."

• • •

The research space in the Boyer Building was a big improvement over the place where he'd done the heart-and-a-half experiments. It was above ground and had windows. There were sinks and benches and wireless internet. Could be worse, he thought. The weather had cleared and he walked home across the campus, beginning a mental list of the students he might ask to come in on the project with him.

Where the sidewalk met the concrete walk that ran to the front door of his apartment block, Leonard Maigrot got out of a black Mercedes with opaqued windows. "Dr. Carras?"

It was a moment before Carras recognized the man. "I'm in no mood for mysteries or mind games," he said.

"May I come in?"

"What for?"

"To talk about the medical matter."

"It won't do any good. My operating privileges at Yale have been suspended. These days I'm just a researcher."

The cold rain had stopped falling but the air was chill. Maigrot rubbed his hands together and blew on them. "Could we do this inside?" he said.

"I told you, I don't see patients at my home. And for the foreseeable future, I won't be seeing patients anywhere at all."

"Doctor..."

"Anything you want to say to me you can say right now. I'm almost certainly going to say no, then you can get back into your nice warm car and leave."

Maigrot pulled one corner of his mouth between his teeth and stared at Carras for a few seconds, his eyes narrowed. Then he said, "All right. My employer is aware of the... difficulties you have experienced the past little while. He still wants to engage your services."

"To do what?"

"I don't know."

Carras blinked. "You don't know?"

"I'm just here to deliver an invitation," Maigrot said. "I assure you it will be worth your while to look into it."

"That's quite an assurance from someone who doesn't know what I'm being invited to do," Carras said. "You say it's a medical matter. Do I assume it's a heart operation?"

"I don't know."

"A transplant?"

Maigrot spread his hands.

"I just told you that I cannot operate..."

"If you would just come with me," Maigrot said. "I have a plane ready to take you to my employer."

"Who is...?" Carras said.

"He'd prefer that he tell you himself."

"I'm really not in the mood for games, Mr. Maigrot. I can recommend a number of excellent surgeons. Arslan Kashmanian in Chicago. Isidore Bretzmeyer in New York."

Maigrot shook his head. "My employer wants you."

"Why?"

"He is convinced you are the right man for the job."

Carras said, "I don't think so."

"If you would just come to see him and let him explain things to you in person."

Carras showed the man the palm of his hand. "No."

Maigrot let out his breath in exasperation. "I must ask you to reconsider," he said. "My employer is prepared to make you a very generous offer. More than you would expect."

"He'll have to find someone else."

"He wants you."

"No. That's final. Good day."

He turned and walked into the apartment building. When he was through the glass outer doors, he looked back. The Mercedes was gone. But before he put the incident out of his mind it occurred to Carras that there had been a difference in Maigrot's approach. The other times, in person and on the phone, the man had acted as if compliance with his employer's wishes was a foregone conclusion. He'd been smug, almost cocky.

This time, he'd been worried.

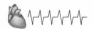

Chapter 4

Leonard Maigrot could have called his employer from the car—it was equipped with a satellite phone with a built-in scrambler function—but he put it off as long as he could, until he was back on board the company jet. The aircraft was a full-sized Boeing 737, reconfigured for the uppermost end of the corporate market and for governments like those of Malaysia and the United Arab Emirates, whose top officials did not have to worry about criticism from the press.

Maigrot was in the plane's lounge, which was the size of a comfortable living room and had ceilings high enough for him to stand without stooping. He got himself a vodka and tonic from the free-standing bar, waving away the attendant, then saying, "I need privacy to make a call."

When the young woman had disappeared into the forward crew area, closing the bulkhead door, Maigrot sat on the ell-shaped couch and drained the vodka. Then he reached for the phone on the built-in coffee table in front of him and touched a button. There were a few seconds' delay as the call was routed through a satellite in geosynchronous orbit above the mid Atlantic, then beamed back down to a yacht moored off a small island in the Bahamas, where Terry Flynnt, chairman of the board and chief executive officer of the

Flynnt Group of companies, was lately spending more and more of his time.

The call was to the private line and the billionaire answered it himself, speaking the single terse syllable that was his name. Maigrot had a clear mental picture of Flynnt at the other end of the connection. The yacht was like the Boeing jet, as big as they came, almost the size of a small cruise ship, and its owner would be in the vast lounge that spanned the entire aft lower deck. The odds were fifty-fifty Flynnt would be grinding away on a computerized exercise cycle, a man well into his sixties who looked closer to forty. If he wasn't on the bike, he'd be in the midst of an endless series of abdominal crunches, or sipping a cocktail of carrot juice, ginkgo biloba and megavitamins.

The sudden fascination with fitness was recent, had started in the past year, and it made Maigrot worry. Men with Flynnt's kind of wealth and power—he was well into the list of the world's twenty richest people—sometimes developed peculiarities that could cause big problems for those who served them.

When he heard Flynnt's voice on the line, Maigrot identified himself and said, "I met with the doctor again."

"What happened?"

Maigrot swallowed. "He won't come."

There was silence.

"He's suspicious," Maigrot said. "He wanted to know what we wanted him to do."

"And you said what?"

"I told him I didn't know, but that it would be worth his while."

"He didn't ask what that meant?"

"He didn't seem interested. He recommended a couple of other doctors, Kashmanian and Bretzmeyer."

"No," Flynnt said. "Carras is the one I want."

"It might help if I could tell him what we want him to do," Maigrot said.

"That's need-to-know, Leonard, and I don't need you to know that."

There was silence on the line. "What do you want me to do?" Maigrot said.

The silence continued, then Flynnt said, "I want to think about it for a while."

"He apparently doesn't respond to money," Maigrot said. "He could make a lot more in private practice than as an academic, but he stays where he is."

Abruptly, Flynnt changed the subject. "What's happening with the Prixcombe placement?"

Maigrot had the facts and figures ready. "We're getting the price we expected—ten per cent below tomorrow's market close—so say eighty-two fifty a share, and he'll take the whole one-point-two million."

"Good. Terms?"

"Straight cash transfer through his Zurich bank to the Caymans account. Should be wrapped by end of business day after tomorrow."

"Good enough," Flynnt said. "And you're feeling out the Singapore group?"

Maigrot said, "We're talking by phone in the morning, our time."

"What's your sense of them?"

"They're pretty hard-ass, even for overseas Chinese. But if I had to bet, I'd lay even money they'll take a million-plus of the preferred shares at about the same price Henri Prixcombe is paying, maybe a point or two less."

"Okay, good."

Maigrot waited to see if anything more was coming. He would have very much liked to know why his boss was having him sell substantial blocks of Flynnt Group shares at under-market prices, and assemble the proceeds into a massive pool of cash and short-term bonds in a numbered account in the Cayman Islands. It had been Maigrot's major occupation for the past three weeks.

But Terry Flynnt never gave out unnecessary information. The silence crackled on the line until Flynnt said, "Something else?"

There was something else. Maigrot shifted a little even though the jet's couch gave superb comfort to his soft buttocks. "Victor Whitehall," he said.

"What about him?"

"He's moving against us. I'm hearing things. He's got us in his sights."

Flynnt said, "It doesn't matter right now."

"I think he's angling for another seat on the board. If he gets it..."

Flynnt said, "That's a big if. Right now, I got bigger ifs to think about. Take the plane to New York then call me once you've talked to Singapore."

"Yes, sir," Maigrot said, but Flynnt was already gone.

• • •

Twelve hundred miles south-southeast of where Maigrot sat worrying about his employer's mental health, Terry Flynnt drained another tumblerful of the fortified juice. He swung his muscular leg over the seat of the Lifestyle 800, slipped his feet into the pedal straps and began to turn the flywheel housed beneath the machine's seat.

A custom-made hardwood rack next to the bike held a number of files. Flynnt took one and spread it open on a matching wooden lectern above the machine's handlebars. He already knew the contents of the dossier, which he had had Maigrot assemble from materials provided by a private research consultancy that specialized in background checks on key personnel. It was everything that could be gathered on Athan Carras, from his formal resume to recent tabloid smears, including the *People* profile, abstracts of the more than two hundred scientific papers he had authored, and even a review of the film *A Thousand Ships*, in the *Yale Daily News* of twenty-three years ago, in which the reviewer, then known as Ath Carras, declared the movie's lead actress to be the most beautiful woman since Helen of Troy.

Flynnt worked the cycle up to a cruising speed that he found comfortable, though it would have soon had a recreational cyclist half his age gasping for oxygen. For the umpteenth time, he immersed himself in the life of Dr. Athan Carras.

• • •

Two weeks after the suspension of his operating privileges, Carras had a thought that surprised him.

It had been two weeks in which nobody had called him in the middle of the night, rousing him out of deep sleep or dream state with some emergency that had to be dealt with right now and correctly, lest someone die.

For two weeks he hadn't had to stand in one spot for eight hours so that afterwards his calf muscles ached like a marathon runner's and woke him out of sleep with unbearable cramps. For two weeks he'd been able to let his brain focus on a professional issue that did not have to be solved soon if not immediately—with life or death in the balance—but could be examined at length and leisure.

The surprising thought, which came as he was shaving at 8:30 a.m.—a time when he would normally be in an operating room with a half hour's work already behind him—was that maybe Cory Goldenberg's death and its sequelae hadn't led to such a bad outcome after all.

People had often said to him that he might be working too hard, or too much. But the words had never really penetrated. It was as if he could understand the meaning of the phrase on some surface level, but was never able to connect the sense of it to any kind of deep understanding of who he was and how he fitted into his own life.

Of course, he hadn't worked steadily, day in and day out, for the twenty-odd years since he'd completed his surgical residency, nor even for the nine years since the break-up of his marriage. There had been vacations—but they had been busy vacations: cycling across France and Germany, mountain climbing in the Alps, a canoeing trip down the Mackenzie River in Canada's high arctic.

And sometimes, in the middle of wherever he was, his pager would beep and he would soon be on a jet heading back to New Haven, because somebody needed his skills. He couldn't recall ever being deeply disappointed at being summoned back to the OR. A beeper call might as well have been a post-hypnotic suggestion, the kind that stage hypnotists implant in volunteers from the audience so that when they hear a particular sound they quack like a duck. The hapless victim never seems to find it strange that he is quacking;

the action takes place at a level of consciousness that is insulated from the normal process of day to day life.

It was a simple thought that surprised Carras. It came as he was scraping away his whiskers because he was shaving in the usual way, quickly swiping the double blade through the lather as if he was in time trials for an Olympic event. But then, as he rinsed the razor under the sink faucet, he stopped and looked at himself in the mirror and said, "What's your hurry?"

It occurred to him that speed shaving was how he did every mundane action, as if life was something he had to get out of the way as quickly as possible so that he could get to the truly important part of the day, which would be either preparing to cut someone open or actually doing so.

"Fact is," he told his reflection, "you don't have to hurry the shave or gulp the breakfast or hustle over to the med center like a speed walker." The three graduate students he had engaged were competently setting up the lab and arranging for the first batch of experimental animals. Carras's major task of the day was to meet with them and discuss the schedule of activities he had asked the senior assistant to prepare.

After that, his only responsibility was to work on the draft of a presentation he would deliver to a conference of cardiologists and cardiothoracic surgeons in Miami in a few days. The booking had been made months before when Carras and the organizers had expected that the subject of his talk would be the heart-and-a-half operation, which would then be beginning human trials.

The Goldenberg case had derailed that plan, but Carras would still appear at the conference. He would talk about his new research initiative, deep hypothermic cardiac arrest, which by then ought to have received the major grant from the Fallon Foundation. Charlie Vance was keeping tabs on the grant application, which was being fast-tracked through the evaluation process.

The Miami conference appearance would confirm that Carras had lost no stature among his peers. Tabloids and TV and even the *New York Times* had played the heart-and-a-half story for its sensational potential, but America's heart specialists knew the significance of Cory Goldenberg's self-dosing with coumadin. Within the profession, Carras was seen as a victim of media-fed hysteria and Miami would be an important step on his return to a normal life.

But do I want to return to that life? he asked himself as he strolled to his lab in the Boyer Building. It was another surprising question. And there was another surprise when he looked for an answer and found that it was: *I'm not sure.*

He met with his student assistants and found everything under control. He worked on his draft presentation for a while then went over to Saybrook College to have lunch with Charlie Vance.

"All seems to be well with your grant," Vance said. "I talked to Thorsteinson on the review committee, and he said they were bending a few procedural rules. You should have unofficial word before Miami."

"Good news," Carras said.

"How are you getting there? I could give you a lift."

Vance had a pilot's license and was rated for both visual and instrument flying. Carras had been up with him in his Cessna 182, had even held the yoke and worked the rudder pedals, but he didn't like being up that high in a craft that sometimes bounced on air currents and thermals like a kid's kite. "No, thanks. I'll stick to jets," he said.

"Getting there is half the fun," Vance said.

"Not getting there at all is what bothers me." Carras was reminded of something. "Speaking of being bothered," he said, "I've had a couple of visits from a mysterious man with an even more mysterious employer who wants to hire me for some unspecified purpose." He described the two meetings with Leonard Maigrot then fished in his pocket and found the man's card.

Vance examined it. "Manhattan area code," he said.

"I figured out that much for myself," Carras said.

Vance took out his cell phone and punched in a number. A few seconds later he said, "Mike, Charlie Vance. You know a guy called Leonard Maigrot?" He listened for a moment then said, "Well, could you check him out, see if anybody knows who he is and who he works for? Not looking to hire him— it's a private matter."

He closed the phone and told Carras that Mike was a corporate headhunter who specialized in high flyers in the New York business establishment. "I figure whoever the mystery boss is, he's private sector. If he was government, ours or somebody else's, this Maigrot guy would probably have let you know."

Vance's phone rang. It was Mike from New York. Vance listened and Carras saw his eyebrows go up. When he closed the phone again, Carras said, "Well?"

"Leonard Maigrot is an executive vice president at the Flynnt Group of companies. But what he really is is the personal assistant to Terry Flynnt."

"Who's Terry Flynnt?" Carras said.

Vance shook his head and poured more wine. "You do live a sheltered life, don't you?" he said. "Terry Flynnt is a self-made billionaire. His companies produce a lot of things that go into various kinds of military hardware."

Carras lifted his refilled glass and drank. "Never heard of him."

"You've heard about his son—I can't remember the name—but he's that playboy race driver who married the supermodel a couple of years back."

That one almost rang a bell for Carras, but he couldn't quite get a grip on it. He shook his head. "What does he want with me?"

Vance shrugged. "From what you tell me, the only person who can answer that question is Terry Flynnt. Why don't you go and ask him?"

Carras thought about it, then he said, "Nah. Chances are, he wants me to operate on him."

"Well, Ath, that is what you do."

"Is it?" Carras said. "I don't know any more."

"Come on, man," Vance said, "Cory Goldenberg's death was not your fault. Don't tell me you're afraid to get back up on the horse."

"I don't know. I don't think it's about being afraid. Maybe I'm just starting to wonder, is this still what I want to do?"

Vance widened his eyes and blinked ostentatiously. "Am I hearing the gentle hum of a mid-life crisis?" he said.

"No," Carras said. "At least I don't think so. Maybe it's just time for a change."

"Ath," said his friend, "growing a beard is a change. Taking up stamp collecting is a change. Giving up surgery, that sounds more like a full-blown revolution."

Carras said nothing, just looked at his hands. "I don't know," he said.

"I'll tell you what I think, since you ask."

"I don't recall asking," Carras said.

"Must've slipped your mind," Vance said. "Anyway, I think you do have some problems over Cory's death. You've lived your entire life by a pretty rigid code of ethics—my word is my bond, that kind of thing. I don't think you've ever stepped over the line." He gave Carras his best impression of Jack Nicholson waiting for an answer.

"I guess not."

"But with Cory, you broke the rules..."

"Technically," Carras said.

"Technically, schmechnically," Vance said. "You broke the rules and the patient died. Maybe you're worried you'll do it again."

"I'm not worried I'll do it again."

Vance looked over at another table where a quartet of English professors was apparently waging a battle over deconstructionism. Their voices were rising. "Do you remember the subject of my master's thesis?" he asked.

"I never read it," Carras said.

"You and thousands more," Vance said. "It was on the influences of Puritan thinking in the development of the American ethical sense."

"Are you about to call me a Puritan? I'd better pour some more wine."

"One of the weaknesses of the Puritan frame of reference is an all-or-nothing mind set."

"Uh huh," said Carras, sipping the wine.

"A Puritan doesn't give in and doesn't compromise. He can't," Vance said.

"Do you know why?"

"For fear of going to hell?"

"For fear of going to hell with the lid off," Vance said, "of going hog wild. Puritans saw themselves as powder kegs of suppressed passions, all the temptations the devil put in their way. They were afraid that if they gave an inch, the floodgates would open and all hell would pour out of them. Any retreat meant the end of their control and that meant the end of the world."

"I'm no Puritan," Carras said. "I bet I've had more women than you." He didn't mention that he'd had most of them before he married Beth. Since the divorce, there had been relatively few relationships, and none that had lasted.

"We're not talking sexual mores, *amigo*. We're talking about where you keep your sense of self-identity," Vance said. "I see you as a Puritan because of your pride."

That took Carras aback. "I thought Puritans were humble folks, went around in simple black clothing, no fancy gew-gaws."

Vance shook his head. "That's the Hollywood version. The reality is that those folks formed the most disciplined army since the Roman legions. They waged war against the king of England a hundred and fifty years before the rest of us did. And after they whupped him, they cut off his head."

"And that's how you see me?"

"If I thought that was all you were, I'd run a mile every time I saw you," Vance said. "You'd be a monster. What I see in you, let's call it a tendency."

"A tendency toward what?"

"Towards that all-or-nothing, victory-or-death kind of thinking."

"I let Auldfield have his victory. I didn't throw myself on my sword."

"You let Boner win an inch so you could take a mile," Vance said. "You held the moral high ground. Everybody who's anybody knows that you did the right thing, that Goldenberg's death was his own fault, that Boner made you jump through absurd hoops. You let him win every battle, but you won the war."

Carras poured a third glass of the wine and sipped it. "I'm just a guy who fixes hearts, Charlie. I don't fight wars."

"I hope not," said Vance. "People get hurt in wars."

"Have some more wine," Carras said.

The conversation moved on, but that afternoon, as he worked on his presentation to the Miami conference, Carras thought about what his friend had said. Was he an all-or-nothing kind of guy? Was that why he had not been able to handle a marriage and fatherhood plus a career, although most of his colleagues managed to do both?

• • •

It was nine-thirty in the morning of the day he was to fly to Miami. At ten a.m., Karen would drive him to the Tweed-New Haven airport to catch the New York shuttle, giving him plenty of time to clear security at La Guardia and connect with the mid-afternoon flight to the south. His suitcase was in the trunk of her car and he was in his office putting the finishing touches to his presentation when she buzzed him. "Charlie Vance," she said.

"I'm at the airport," his friend said. "I thought I'd give Karl Thorsteinson one last call before taking off."

"And?" Carras said, his fingers working the built-in mouse of his laptop, scrolling down through the text of his talk.

"Something's hinky about the grant," Vance said.

Vance was the only person Carras knew who would use a word like hinky. He kept scrolling. "What do you mean, hinky? What did he say?"

"He wouldn't talk to me about it. Just said, 'I'm sorry, it's out of my hands' and hung up. Now I can't get him back."

Carras's fingers froze on the mouse. "What does that mean?"

"I don't know," Vance said. "Karl sounded upset, but I don't know what the hell's going on."

"What about your other contact on the review committee?"

"McIvor?" Vance said. "I tried him. His assistant said he'd have to call me back, but I think he was just ducking."

Carras said, "What the hell's going on? I'm going to Miami to announce the research project. If there's no grant, there's no announcement."

"I don't know what to tell you," Vance said.

Carras snapped the laptop shut. "Well, they can't hide behind their phones and assistants in Miami," he said. "They're both going to be there for the conference. I'll track them down and ask them face to face."

"That's a plan," Vance said. "Look, I've got to get into the air. I'll see you down there tonight."

"You're on."

• • •

The woman in the seat beside him wanted to talk.

"Will you be in Miami long?" she asked, as the plane backed away from the gate.

"Just a couple of days."

"Business or pleasure?"

"A conference," he said.

"You look familiar," she said. "Have we met?"

His stint as America's bogey man must be drawing to an end. She hadn't recognized Dr. Death. "I don't think so," he said.

"What do you do?" she said, and he caught the quick look at the naked ring finger of his left hand.

"I'm sorry, but I have to work," Carras said. He opened his briefcase and got out the text of his presentation to the medical conference. If he wasn't getting the grant—and how the hell did that happen?—he'd have to rewrite most of it. The final draft led off with a gracious thank-you to the Fallon Foundation for its assistance. That had to come out. He had also phrased much of the body of the text in straight declarative statements, outlining a full program that began with a review of the existing literature, which was skimpy, then moving to animal studies and ultimately going to trials on human volunteers.

Now all of that certainty was reduced to mere proposal. Instead of telling his assembled peers what he would soon be doing, he could only talk about what he would like to do, if given the chance. Instead of opening their eyes to a bold new direction in surgery, he would be letting them in on his hopes.

He made the changes and returned the papers to his briefcase. He still had the original presentation on his notebook computer, complete with Power-Point slides as illustrations. If he could talk to Thorsteinson and McIvor in Miami perhaps he could yet turn this around.

He was puzzled by what Charlie Vance had said: Yale had been putting its full weight behind him, or so he had been led to believe. Now he wondered if there had been another campaign being waged against him. Had James Bonar Auldfield been calling in favors, twisting the arms of old frat brothers, determined that having got Carras down once he would make sure his rival never got back up?

When Vance had first proposed that he research DHCA, it had seemed like just something to do—something worthwhile, but still just a time-filler until he got back to the real work of opening and closing chests. But something had happened in the intervening weeks, Carras realized, because now the thought of losing the project was pulling a feeling out of his psychological basement, and the feeling could only be described as panic.

He was a surgeon, first and foremost, and everything else in his life came after—way after. That's what had cost him his marriage and his son. Beth had explained it to him in plain terms across the kitchen table on one of those rare Saturdays when he was actually home instead of at the hospital, or at some medical conference, or off on some exchange program teaching foreign doctors how to do the things that he did. She was not prepared to remain the wife of a man who did not put her and their child first above all things. Beth Cavendish was not born to be anyone's second choice.

When they married, she hadn't realized that Athan Carras already had a wife. He was indissolubly wed to his work. It hadn't been a lifelong calling; he hadn't even thought of medicine until he won a place in med school. It was all just more interesting things to learn, another game of the mind, until a professor handed him a scalpel for the first time and told him to open up a living human being.

The operation had only been a baby step: an abdominal incision, no bones to saw through, a nice big cyst that was easy to isolate and remove. But as Carras had watched his own hand making the cut, steady and smooth, as he had seen the layers of skin part and beneath them the beautiful intricacies of organs, blood vessels and tissues, a window had opened up in his soul and light had flooded in.

He had never known such excitement before, a sense that of all the places in the universe where he might have been, and of all the things that he might have been doing, he had unexpectedly found himself in exactly the right place, doing just what he was made to do. In the OR, he was whole, he was complete, he was perfect.

Which meant that, outside that brightly lit small room, he would always be incomplete. Even when he was with the woman he loved and the child they had made together, he was only a pale copy of that bigger, fuller Athan Carras who somehow appeared whenever he walked into the OR. And Beth Cavendish was not content to live with a mere shadow.

She had tried to make it work. She began with reasonable suggestions: let's make sure we set aside enough time for ourselves; how about you take a couple of weeks off in July and we'll go somewhere; it would be good if you could spend more time with Costas, maybe take him to tee-ball.

It had ended at the dining room table, the bright summer sun coming in through the tall windows, when he announced that he would be spending three weeks in Cardiff teaching at the University of Wales, and she announced that when he came back she would not be there. Nor would his son.

"He'd be better off not having a father than to have one who brushes past him on the way to something more interesting," she said. "And I've taken all of this that I intend to take."

She had tried everything she could think of, but sharing a life with him was like living with an addict. She knew he had always loved his work, but now it seemed to her that he craved it the way a drunk craved his bottle, or a junkie his needle. And it was getting worse.

"I don't think you can help it," she said. "Or maybe you just don't want to help it. Either way, it's over."

It wasn't a particularly acrimonious divorce. The financial arrangements weren't a problem—Beth had inherited more money than Carras could have earned in a decade. At the end of it, she said, "You've made your choice, and I've made mine. I just hope, for your sake, that you don't wake up one day and find that you've thrown away a wife and family for something that turned out in the end to be not worth it."

Now, sitting in business class on yet another jet taking him to yet another conference, Athan Carras realized that he was afraid—deeply afraid—that Beth had been right. The outcome that she had warned him about had suddenly popped up in his path. And if his best friend was also right, if he was the rigid personality that insightful Charlie Vance saw him to be, he might no longer be able to do the work that told him who he was.

But if he was no longer a surgeon, what was he? He remembered reading a book that his father had given him, a biography of Alexander the Great, the greatest Greek of them all. Alexander had conquered all that there was to conquer, marching to the ends of the world, winning every battle. But then, on the shores of the farthest river, he sat down and wept because beyond it there was nothing left for him to master, nothing that would allow him to go on being what he was meant to be. What he needed to be.

"I need..." he said, and when the woman beside him put down her historical romance and said, "I beg your pardon?" he was startled to find that he had spoken aloud.

"Sorry, just thinking out loud," he said, but the words had come from some profound part of him. *I need,* he said in the privacy of his own mind, waiting to hear, wanting to hear, his deeper self finish the thought. But the conclusion didn't come, only the recognition by the part of him that waited for the answer that he needed something to make him whole again.

• • •

The conference was in the new Loews Hotel, the first luxury hotel built in Miami's South Beach in decades, incorporating a gleaming new eighteen-story tower with a complete refurbishment of the old art-deco classic, the St. Moritz. Carras caught the hotel's shuttle bus from the airport and checked in just before five p.m. Registration didn't begin until seven, but there were already a few early birds whose faces he recognized from previous gatherings. He avoided talking to them and went straight to his room overlooking the gentle rollers on Miami's endless silver beach.

He didn't bother to empty his suitcase but got on the phone to the front desk and asked to be connected to the rooms of Karl Thorsteinson and Alan McIvor. Neither man had checked in yet, so he left messages asking each to call his cell phone number. He made sure the battery was fully charged before going down to the palm-filled lobby. He found a corner where he had a good view of the doors where the airport shuttle arrived. He would wait, and eventually he would see one of them come in. Then he would casually walk over and begin a conversation.

He felt vulnerable and exposed, even in the relatively secluded corner. He practiced staring into the middle distance so as not to catch the eye of anyone who might want to come over and go through the long-time-no-see ritual.

But whenever a shuttle pulled in, which seemed to be about every twenty minutes, he locked his eyes onto the main doors and held them there until he was sure neither of his targets had appeared.

He had just dismissed the fourth shuttle's complement of incoming guests, when a woman's voice beside him said, "May I ask a favor?"

It was an oddly familiar voice, a smoky, warm contralto. He recognized it right away as a voice he had heard many times, but it was as if the memory was the recalling of something that was not from real life, but out of a dream. When he turned and looked up, all at once the sense of dreaminess seemed completely appropriate.

He bounced to his feet, then blinked and opened his mouth only to find that nothing was coming out of it. Finally, he managed to say, "You're Hilary Cartiere."

"Yes, I know," she said.

Carras felt heat in his face. He hadn't blushed since high school, but he could feel the capillaries in his face filling and opening. "You wanted to ask a favor?" he said.

She smiled—which is to say the sun came up and filled his world with a golden light—and said, "May I sit with you? I have to wait for someone for a few minutes, and when I'm on my own sometimes men can be..." she motioned perfectly with a perfect hand "...a nuisance. Especially men at conventions."

Carras managed not to stammer as he said, "Please," then racked his mind for something witty to say, some well crafted line that a suave hero would toss off in a sophisticated movie that starred Hilary Cartiere.

It ought to have been easy. He'd seen every film she'd ever made, seen each one more than once, many of them more than twice. And from the age of nineteen, he'd seen her in more of his dreams than he could have counted.

He sat down beside her and thought it would be a good idea to say, "My name is Athan Carras."

• • •

Later that evening, he and Charlie Vance had dinner in the old St. Moritz dining room, now splendidly refurbished like something from a 1930s movie. Carras couldn't help going on about the twenty minutes he had spent talking with the most beautiful woman on earth.

They had sat in the encouraged closeness of a love seat, the privacy sheltered by a vast tropical fern, their heads inclined together, their voices low. Twice, she had laughed, a musical sound yet full of earthy undertones. Once, she had touched his hand; it sent a shock through his being that he hadn't experienced since the first time he had slipped his hand inside a girl's clothes and felt the mystery of the flesh.

"She said it must be amazing to touch someone's living heart," he told

Vance. He kept seeing her in his head: her eyes were gray, flecked with gold. She must be pushing fifty, he knew, but even at this close a distance, he wouldn't have taken her for more than thirty-five. Her muscle tone was superb, the flesh along her jaw and under her throat as firm as that of a woman half her age. If there had been any evidence of a plastic surgeon's craft, his expert eye would have caught it.

Charlie Vance said something, and Carras realized he had drifted away. "Sorry, what?"

Vance said, "I asked you what did you say when she said the thing about touching hearts?"

"I said, 'I think you've touched more hearts than I have,'" Carras said. It sounded corny, telling it to Vance, but when he'd said it to Hilary Cartiere, he'd been thrilled that she responded with a widening of her eyes and a subtle repositioning of her sculpted brows. It was exactly the same expression in *Moonfire* when Nick Nolte told her that he was leaving his wife to be with her.

"So she asked what brought me to Miami Beach," he told Vance, "and I told her about the presentation and the research project into DHCA."

He didn't tell his friend that he had gone on at some length, validating the observation frequently made by female stand-up comedians that what men want most is to sit with a beautiful woman who's dying to hear them talk about their work.

He had gone on and on about suspended animation. But, amazingly she had hung on his every word, saying, "Fascinating," and "I'd no idea," and "Please tell me more."

And he had done so, at length, talking not just about the scientific value of DHCA, but about how much the work meant to him personally. He opened himself to her, revealing feelings he was only just coming to recognize in himself, baring his heart as he had never done to anyone—not to Charlie Vance at times like this, when a bottle of good Bordeaux was sacrificing itself between them, not even to Beth over the kitchen table in the long ago.

But he felt that Hilary Cartiere understood, probably not all the details, but certainly what the work meant to him. More than that, he felt that she understood him, that she clearly saw Athan Carras for who he was and even better, that she liked what she saw. He couldn't help making a comparison with the years with Beth. Maybe it hadn't been all his fault, he thought. Maybe he just hadn't found the right woman.

"It was amazing, Charlie," he told his friend, feeling the wine warming his cheeks. "It was like we'd known each other for years."

More than that, it was as if they had liked each other for years. All those hours spent in movie theaters and later in front of a television watching her on video, he had felt that she was the perfect woman. And now it seemed that she was perfect for him.

He didn't tell Vance that at some point in the conversation beneath the spreading fern, he had seen Karl Thorsteinson across the lobby. And when he looked, there was Alan McIvor. He saw them meet and talk and walk away together, but Carras made no move to follow them. He was talking with Hilary Cartiere.

"What was she doing in Miami?" Vance asked.

"It was kind of vague," Carras said. "Some meetings, I think about a part in a movie."

"Been quite a while since she made a film."

"I told her it would be great to see her in something like *Five Bullets*," Carras said. "She was totally amazing in that."

He was glad of the wine and the warmth it brought to his cheeks because he did not want Charlie Vance to know that he was blushing at the memory of how he had gone on and on about the famous scene in that movie where she goes to plead with the crooked senator, and he tells her to take off her blouse. Carras had found himself burbling like a sophomore. "I'm sorry," he told her.

"It's all right," she said. "That scene made my career. In this business, you use what you've got." For a moment, he saw something else in her eyes, but then she had reached over and touched his hand, her fingers warm on his skin, and said, "I'm going to have to go now."

"I hope I didn't offend..."

Now she squeezed his hand. "No, but my car has arrived."

Carras looked up to see a huge man with coffee-colored skin coming toward them. The man was about fifty, wearing a well tailored blue suit. He had the calm face of a preacher but moved with an economy of motion that suggested that the body under the suit was hard and superbly coordinated. Carras thought he looked like one of those professional soldiers who retired to become bodyguards.

Hilary stood up as he neared them and Carras rose with her. She made introductions, and Carras learned that the man's name was Isaac Dumoulin. More than that he did not learn, except that the man's gaze was impassive and his handshake implied controlled strength.

"It's been a pleasure to meet you," Hilary said.

"Perhaps we'll see each other again," Carras said, but her only answer was a nod accompanied by a shrug. The other man inclined his head in the briefest motion and led her away.

Carras watched her all the way to the door and it was only when she was gone from his sight that he realized he should have asked where she was staying, gotten a phone number, something, anything to allow him to follow up. *Dumb as a teenager*, he castigated himself.

He made a circuit of the hotel's public areas, looking for Thorsteinson and McIvor, but they were nowhere to be seen. He went to his room and phoned them again, but with no more success than the first time. Then Vance called and he went down to dinner.

Vance shared out the last of the Bordeaux. "I wonder what happened to Thorsteinson and McIvor?" he said.

"I don't know," said Carras. "Let's order another bottle."

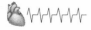

Chapter 5

Before eight a.m., Athan Carras had finished breakfast in the hotel restaurant. He lingered over his coffee, watching for either of the two review committee members, but they didn't appear.

After eight-thirty, Charlie Vance came in and sat down. "Anything?" Carras said.

Vance poured the last of the coffee from the carafe and sipped it. Then he put the cup down and chewed on his inner lip while his brow furrowed. "I found out what room Thorsteinson is in and went and knocked on his door," he said. "He was having breakfast with McIvor and Yussuf Mahmoud. Do you know him?"

"No," Carras said.

"Me neither, but he's on the review committee, too."

"So what happened. What did they say?"

"It's more what they didn't say," Vance said. "They wouldn't talk about it. It's like they're all ashamed—like some Victorian family that's bundled the dotty old auntie off to the funny farm and nobody's supposed to mention it. It's weird."

"From the outside it may be weird," said Carras. "From where I sit it's infuriating."

"One thing," Vance said. "Thorsteinson showed me to the door, very gentlemanly."

"Gosh, how nice."

"But when we got there, he sort of whispered, 'Tell him it's only temporary—not a refusal, a delay.'"

"What the hell does that mean? Why a delay?"

"That's what I asked him," Vance said, "but all I got was a head shake and the door closed in my face."

Carras tossed his napkin onto the table. He had already signed for the check. "What's the room number? I'm going to hunt them up."

"They'll be gone," Vance said. "They're hiding. They won't show their faces where you can see them until you've made your presentation."

"What the hell, Charlie." Carras stared at the crumpled napkin as if an answer might be lurking somewhere in its folds.

"I don't know, Ath. All I can tell you is, roll with it till we see what it is."

Carras stood up. "You coming?"

"No, I'm going to make some more calls, see if I can reach some people upstream from the review committee, find out what happened."

"Okay."

"But I'm not holding out much hope. My friend, you've been nobbled—and from a great height. Guys like Thorsteinson and McIvor don't cave easily."

"Auldfield?" Carras said.

Vance looked up at him. "Not unless he's got a doting uncle with a senator in his pocket. It would take at least that kind of power."

• • •

The conference's keynote speaker was scheduled for nine, and Carras was to follow with the first presentation at nine-fifteen. He would have to deliver the text he had rewritten on his laptop instead of reading from the original print-out, now much scratched and slashed. He wasn't confident that he could reorder the PowerPoint slides to match the changes in the text—Karen handled that kind of thing—and rather than risk making a mess of the graphics he opted to leave the big screen behind the speaker's podium a blank blue. He felt a flash of anger at the mess somebody was making of his plans, but he pushed it away.

Carrying the laptop, he left the restaurant and crossed the lobby, slipping into the flow of name tag-bearing doctors that was heading toward the main ballroom. When he reached the big double doors a hand touched his arm and a woman's voice said, "Dr. Carras, I've been looking for you."

She was from the program committee, one of those efficient young professionals who make conventions work. She steered him toward the dais at the

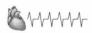

front of the ballroom. Most of the floor space was taken up with rows of chairs, now filling up with medical people. In the crowd were several senior practitioners in cardiothoracic surgery, Carras's peers and colleagues and— some of them—his rivals for pre-eminence in one of the profession's most difficult arts.

The young woman—her lapel tag said her name was Birgit—led him to the front row of chairs which had colored index cards on the seats identifying them as reserved for speakers. When he sat, she presented both palms toward him like a kindergarten teacher silently urging a rambunctious child to stay where he was put. Carras turned in his seat and looked out across the sea of faces. He automatically acknowledged smiles and nods from acquaintances who caught his eye, but he didn't see Thorsteinson or McIvor.

He heard an electronic hiss, followed by an amplified voice saying, "Ladies and gentlemen, doctors, I want to welcome you all to this conference..." Time's up, he thought and turned to face the podium.

The keynoter was given by David Bardoloni, president of the American Heart Association, an accomplished speaker who was usually a pleasure to listen to. Carras heard the audience laugh a number of times, but none of Bardoloni's witticisms penetrated and for all he knew the man had been speaking Urdu. Then he heard his own name coming through the speakers. He got up and went to the podium.

Under ordinary circumstances, Carras was a good speaker. He hadn't had the jitters in front of an audience for a long time. But when he placed the laptop on the podium and adjusted the mike, he saw that his hands were actually shaking. It had been a long time since he had had to call upon the lessons he'd taken in public speaking, back when he had been a young doctor. He remembered them now, and consciously fixed his attention on a point in the air midway back above the crowd. He took a long, slow breath, in and out, and got started.

"Let me tell you about a man who woke up in the morgue in Cairo, Egypt, a couple of years ago," he said. "They had pronounced him dead and put him in a coffin twelve hours before. There shouldn't have been enough air in the coffin to keep him alive that long, but fortunately for Mr." —he looked at his notes to read the name—"Abdel-Sattar Abdel-Salam Badawi, they put the coffin in the morgue refrigerator.

"He woke up in darkness, and reached out. His hands pushed the coffin lid away and he started shouting. The morgue attendants came, and one of them was so shocked he collapsed and died of a heart attack."

There was a titter from someone in the crowd, immediately suppressed. "Let me tell you about another case," Carras continued. He spun the laptop's mouse and noticed that the tremor was gone from his hand. His nerves were back in their proper places. He knew the material, and knew it was good. From here on in, it should go well.

He told them about the Harrison family, a mom and dad with two children, a girl of eight and a six-year-old boy. They'd been driving home from a winter outing with the kids when they hit a patch of ice on Route 34 just outside Derby. The van skidded off the road and into a river. They were in the water—under the water—a long time. When the police divers pulled them out, they were stone cold dead.

"No pulse, no respiration, body temperature eighteen degrees Celsius," said Carras. "Luckily, though, they came into Yale Med Center at the end of the surgical shift. It was four in the afternoon, all the surgical teams were still on the premises and the ORs were empty.

"So we took them into Rooms 14, 15, 16 and 17, all in a row, and put them on heart-lung bypass machines. I did the father. We began rewarming the bodies by warming their blood with the machines and recirculating it back through their systems. At thirty-two degrees, each heart started beating spontaneously. At thirty-six degrees, we weaned them from bypass. They were alive."

The story had a bittersweet ending. Because their bodies were larger, the parents had cooled more slowly after the icy water had invaded their lungs. Their internal organs had had time to deteriorate, especially their brains. They lived, but only technically, for several days after reanimation, then died without regaining consciousness.

The children's smaller bodies, however, had cooled more rapidly. They made a good recovery and showed no mental or physical impairment, though they had been stone-cold dead for almost two hours before their hearts had begun to beat again in the ORs. They went to live with their mother's sister and her husband, who were unable to have children of their own.

"The incident set me thinking," Carras said. "As you know, it is routine in expert centers to use heart-lung machines to cool cardiac surgery patients during operations on the aorta. I myself have used the technique over 1000 times. If the body is cooled rapidly, the organs shut themselves down as though someone has pushed a biological pause button"—he gave the phrase particular emphasis, because he was proud of it—"until warm blood starts the body up again."

He paused and looked around the room. "Ladies and gentlemen, doctors, I believe that in developing the technique of deep hypothermic circulatory arrest, DHCA, we have barely opened a door. Beyond that door may lie the suspended animation of human beings for prolonged, even indefinite, periods."

Carras had given enough presentations to know that his bold statement should be followed by a murmur of reaction in the crowd. But he didn't expect to hear a harsh voice somewhere in the anonymity of the audience call out, "Hogwash!"

He looked to see if anyone was getting to his feet to challenge him. He'd seen Arslan Kashmanian in the crowd, with whom he had crossed swords before, although he thought Chicago's top cardiothoracic surgeon was too much a professional of the old school to interrupt a colleague with blatant rudeness. But there was Kashmanian in the second row, turning his head with many others in the audience trying to locate the heckler.

Carras ignored the outburst and went on. But he noticed that the tremor had returned to his fingers. "As you know,"—there was a sudden dryness in his throat, and he coughed and started again—"As you know, it is common practice to use DHCA to cool patients so that we can work in the body's high-rent districts—the center of the aortic arch or the depths of the brain. I am of the opinion..."

"Science fiction!" said a voice in the crowd.

"Beam me up, Scotty!" said another.

Now the audience was more interested in discovering who the hecklers were than in listening to what Carras had to say. Still, no one was getting up to give him an argument.

"I would be happy to debate my views with anyone who would care to offer an opposing argument," he said, meanwhile thinking, *Could I sound more stuffy?* "But I would appreciate the courtesy of first being allowed to state them."

There were no more outbursts. But it didn't matter; Carras had lost the initiative. His original text had led up to an announcement that he would be conducting a major research project to extend the bounds of DHCA beyond conventional limits, to achieve the protracted suspended animation of a human being. But with the grant withheld, all he could talk about were the small, informal experiments he had done with mice and laboratory rats, cooling them and keeping them suspended for twenty-four hours, after which they ran their mazes and pushed levers to get food pellets as if nothing had happened.

The presentation should have ended with a bold vision of the future; instead, Carras knew, it wimped out with his expression of hope that he would soon be able to mount more far-reaching experiments. There was polite applause, undercut by two or three people in the audience who were deliberately clapping in slow, methodical unison, mocking him from within the concealment of the crowd.

As he stood down from the dais, Carras saw that a couple of doctors he knew were moving to the front as if they wanted to speak with him. Carras was used to being the center of a post-presentation discussion; his talks tended to stimulate minds. But right now, he just wanted out. He waved off the klatch before it could develop, pointing to his watch and miming a phone to his ear as he strode rapidly toward the exit doors.

Before he could get there, a man with a pen and notebook blocked his way, and said, "Just a follow-up question, doctor."

A couple more reporters closed in as soon as Carras stopped moving.

The first man had a red-veined nose and wore a narrow-brimmed straw hat. He said, "This thing you have about freezing people, is that why you call yourself 'The Ice Man?'"

The People profile again. Carras heartily wished he had never opened his mouth to the media. "Let me pass, please," he said.

"Isn't that what you call yourself? Or is it Doctor Ice?" the reporter said. "You don't happen to have on a cape and tights under your suit, do you? With a big capital I on your chest?"

"Are you crazy?" Carras said. "What paper are you with?"

He had raised his voice. Now a couple more media types were zeroing in on the little group, detecting controversy the way sharks scent blood in the water. One of the first three said, "The death of Dr. Cory Goldenberg, was that a result of your bizarre theories?"

"My theories are not bizarre," Carras said. A set of camera lights blazed into his face. "I've got documented..."

"But this whole cryogenics business was exposed as nothing but a scam back in the nineteen-seventies," the reporter said.

"It's not cryogenics. It's cooling, not freezing."

The red nosed man was back at him again, tilting his hat back with one finger. "That business with the family that drowned," he said. "Are you experimenting on people's loved ones after they've passed away? Is this some kind of Frankenstein thing, trying to bring back the dead?"

Carras's mouth fell open. "That's got to be the stupidest question I've ever been asked," he began.

"But I don't hear you answering it."

A microphone appeared under Carras's nose. "Aren't you just seeking notoriety to drum up more business from your celebrity clientele?" said a woman's voice.

Now Carras realized that he was in the center of something he had only seen on TV and in the movies: the feeding frenzy of a hostile media scrum. He did what he had always seen politicians and accused criminals do. He said, "No comment," inserted himself between two of the reporters and walked away. But the pack went with him, and the questions never stopped.

"What are you afraid of, doctor?"

"Why are you running?"

"Have you experimented on the dead?"

He made it to the open doorway that led into the hallway, the scrum still at his heels. But as he passed through the opening, Carras scarcely noticed the large dark skinned man with close cropped hair who stepped neatly into his wake and barred the path of the pursuing pack. "Show's over," the man said, and though the voice was soft the reporters stopped as if they had encountered a force field dressed in a gray two-button suit.

The foyer outside the ballroom was almost empty, the elevators not far. Carras fixed his eyes on the elevator doors and kept walking. After a moment, his peripheral vision told him that someone was keeping pace beside him. "No comment," he said again.

"Looks like you could use a friend," said a voice he knew, a warm voice that made him stop and turn. Hilary Cartiere put a hand on his arm and stepped closer, touching her cheek to his. He heard the sound of her lips parting beside his ear.

"Oh, my god," he said. "It's you."

"I think you could also use a little vacation from all of this."

"That's for sure," Carras said.

"Then come with me." She shifted her hand so that it was on the back of his upper arm and applied a gentle pressure. They went past the elevators and down a staircase that led to the lobby.

"Where are we going?" Carras said. But it didn't really matter where, what was important was who with? In the conference room, the situation had been out of his control and he'd felt anger and frustration. Now he was in another situation, equally out of his control, but all he felt was the excitement of being with this incredible woman, of moving toward some wonderful adventure.

"Let me surprise you," she said.

"You already have."

They cut across the lobby and went out into the porchere, where they stopped. Carras looked a question at her, and she held up a hand in gesture that said, Wait for it. Less than a minute went by before a limousine pulled up in front of them and the driver, a big man in a gray suit, got out and opened the rear door for them.

"You remember Isaac," Hilary said.

"Good morning, sir" said the chauffeur, and Carras realized that he had just heard the man's voice saying "Show's over," to the media pack upstairs.

"Good morning, Isaac," Carras said. "And thank you for throwing the block."

"My pleasure, sir," said Isaac. He let them get seated then closed the door.

Carras settled back and looked at Hilary. She was still the most beautiful woman on earth. He saw Isaac's head and shoulders appear through the darkened panel between the passenger and driver's compartments, then the car moved smoothly away.

"Where are we going?" Carras asked.

Hilary was reaching into a space built into the side of the limo forward of the rear door. He couldn't help noticing the lines of lithe body. She brought out a bottle of champagne and two frosted flute glasses.

"Paradise," she said.

• • •

Leonard Maigrot was a man with few illusions about himself. He knew he had brains. Put him in a room with a hundred people chosen at random and he could expect to be smarter than at least ninety-eight of them. He knew he had a knack for analyzing people and the relationships between them, especially when those relationships involved power. He had ambition and he had the built-in ruthlessness that should have enabled him to get whatever he wanted. He lacked only the nerve.

He'd known that he was missing some crucial ingredient as far back as the elementary school yard. He could hit smaller kids and it didn't bother him that he was hurting them. But he couldn't bear to be hit. He would avoid fights even against boys he knew he could beat, because the prospect of a fist splitting his own lip or a sneakered foot sinking into his own belly filled him with a feeling that was more sadness than fear. He couldn't stand the thought of it and when some kid was said to be gunning for him he would lie in bed at night with his cold hands clasped between his drawn up thighs, imagining and dreading.

He soon learned that his best strategy was to attach himself to a group of bigger, tougher kids and be the brains of the outfit. Lunch-money protection rackets became much more profitable under his guidance, the money collected through extortion being spun over into a high-school loan sharking set-up that paid real dividends.

If Maigrot had been developing his talents in a suitable environment—like an inner-city barrio—he might have graduated to a career in professional crime. But being raised in the leafy suburbs of Southbury, Connecticut, the son of a successful financial consultant, he went instead to Harvard Business School. In a second year seminar, a classmate summed him up: "All Maigrot wants is to be the biggest flea on the biggest dog." Maigrot did not immediately recognize the description as an insult.

But this morning, as he had listened to Dr. Athan Carras make his presentation and seen him be ambushed by the posse of actors that Maigrot had arranged, he had been worrying that he might be a flea that had chosen the wrong dog.

The business at the surgical conference bothered him: not the disruption of the doctor's performance and the phony hostile media scrum that followed, but the subject of Athan Carras's presentation. In the research package he had put together for Terry Flynnt, the DHCA experiments were only a minor footnote. Essentially, the surgeon was a man who fixed or replaced unhealthy hearts, had been doing it for twenty years, and was one of the best in the world. Maigrot had no idea why his employer had become so fixated on this heart surgeon—Flynnt certainly showed no signs of heart disease—but the executive had assumed it had something to do with cutting and sewing.

Now this suspended animation thing opened up a whole new area of speculation, and Maigrot suspected it was not one that he would enjoy exploring. He was starting to worry that Terry Flynnt might be edging toward that invisible border that separated arrogant business genius from nut case with more money than was good for him.

The boss was showing signs that he might be another Howard Hughes in the making. Maigrot remembered the stories about the reclusive billionaire hiding from germs behind his phalanx of Mormon praetorians, flitting from hotel to hotel and allegedly giving a fortune away to a truck driver who picked him up hitchhiking.

Being tied to such a man was not a future that appealed to Leonard Maigrot. The next stage in his career, as he envisioned it, should have involved his stepping into the CEO slot at one of the key profit centers of the Flynnt Group. Instead, he found himself arranging mind games for a heart surgeon who wanted to put people into cold storage.

Maigrot added Carras's research into suspended animation to the other unusual interests Terry Flynnt had taken up in the past several months, and the total didn't look good. Flynnt had always been healthy, fitter than most his age, but he had never been an ascetic. He had liked a good rare steak and a twelve-year-old scotch. But lately he had given up red meat in favor of tofu and vegetables, and all he drank now was concoctions like the carrot juice and ginkgo biloba.

He'd had a fully equipped gym installed on the yacht, and another one next to his office in Manhattan. He worked out at least two hours every day, and took a slew of vitamins, minerals and nutritional supplements morning and night.

Coincident with the health kick had come the mysterious selling off of blocks of Flynnt Group stock. The shares had come from Flynnt's personal holdings, and the proceeds had created an enormous pool of liquidity at Bank Caribe in the Cayman Islands. Maigrot had tried—to be blunt, he had spied on his boss—to find out what the money and short-term financial instruments, now approaching a billion dollars, were intended for. The most he could discover was that some of the funds had been spent on medical equipment, more on some kind of construction project. But what and where were still as deep a mystery to Maigrot as the big question: why?

Now he saw the inklings of an answer, and the shape of things that might be about to come scared the hell out of him. Could it be that Terry Flynnt was building himself a living mausoleum, a facility where he would lie in suspended animation for a decade or two, until research into stem cells or the human genome came up with a way to let people—some people, that is, some really rich people—tack another thirty or forty vigorous years onto their already extended life spans?

If that was the case, Maigrot doubted that Flynnt would be suspending any of the fleas that relied on him for their hopes and dreams. Like a dog in winter, Flynnt would let his hangers-on face the chilly world all on their own.

Leonard Maigrot had not done that since grade school, and he had no intention of doing it now.

• • •

Carras had flown in private jets many times before, sometimes to harvest hearts, sometimes when wealthy patients had wished to express their gratitude for his saving their lives by offering him a temporary dip in the luxury on which they floated every day. But the Boeing Business Jet—a modified 737—was an order of magnitude more sumptuous than anything he had sampled before. The lounge was the size of a small living room, and there were apparently actual bedrooms at the rear of the plane. He saw no plastic on the walls, only rich wood paneling and what looked like silk wallpaper. The floor was carpeted in a deep burgundy, with a pile thick enough to lose small animals.

Instead of seats, there was an L-shaped couch built around a coffee table of some exotic wood. Hilary led him to it and they sat down, her firm thigh against his. Isaac went forward and through a door. Almost immediately, a blonde young woman came back the other way. She brought glasses and champagne from the bar across the lounge and, after showing Carras and Hilary where seat belts emerged from the furniture, she poured for them and said that they would be taking off immediately. Then she went through the door up forward and left them alone.

"This is... amazing," Carras said. He could feel a big grin splitting his face but he didn't try to control it. This was a miracle and he was just going to enjoy it.

Hilary held out her glass and he touched his to it, the musical clink almost lost in the revving up of the jet's twin engines. The plane rolled smoothly forward and it seemed no more than a minute before they were rushing down the runway and climbing the air. When they heard the undercarriage clunk into the wheel wells beneath their feet, she said, "Now, you were telling me last night about your experiments."

The last thing Carras wanted to talk about this morning was suspended animation. "Never mind that," he said. "Tell me what it's like to be you."

She turned her head a little to one side and gave him a look that he knew he'd seen on a big screen. It had even more impact in real life. "I'm just a woman, you know," she said.

"Oh, yeah," he said. "And the Mona Lisa's just a picture."

"What was that line from *A Thousand Ships?*" she said, "I am a mirror and all men see in me..."

"...the fulfillment of their desires," he finished for her.

"You really are a fan."

"Only your greatest." It was his turn to offer a toast and when their glasses touched he said, "To the most beautiful woman in the world."

She smiled at that, and he wished he could freeze-frame the moment and hold it forever. Then she sipped the champagne and it was gone.

"You said you were in Miami for a meeting about a part. Did it go well? Are you going to be making another picture?"

"It looks that way."

"That would be great. You'd be starring, right?"

Another expression appeared on her face, almost too briefly to register, then she smiled. "That's the deal," she said.

The conversation moved on. He urged her to do the talking, liking the rich timber of her voice. She told him gossip about famous people: a distinguished actor who became a petulant, self-centered schlub if the wrong brand of mineral water was placed in his dressing room; a brilliant director who routinely singled out some supporting player to be the target of his vicious temper; a big-name screenwriter who had created nothing of his own for ten years, only rewriting the work of others, while taking all the credit.

Carras listened, leaning forward when she lowered her voice to impart a confidence, although there was no one there. Ordinarily, he disdained gossip. He remembered a line Charlie Vance had once quoted: People with great minds talk about ideas; those with second-rate minds talk about other people; those with scarcely any minds at all talk about themselves. But he would have listened to Hilary Cartiere read the owner's manual to her DVD player with equally rapt attention.

They had barely reached cruising altitude when he felt the aircraft tilt downward. He looked out the window but saw only sky and sea. He realized he didn't even know what direction they'd been flying. "We haven't gone far," he said.

"It's only about eighty miles from Miami," she said. There was a control panel set into the end of the couch. She pressed a button and the young woman came back to refill her glass. Carras waved the bottle away. He hadn't drunk alcohol this early in the day since he was an undergraduate and he was feeling a definite buzz.

The jet tipped onto its left wing and dropped some more. Carras looked out the window and saw an island shaped like a thickened parenthesis, its coast ringed with white beach and with a low hill at one end. A pane of glass on a building halfway up the hill threw a dazzle of sun into his eyes, then the plane continued to turn and he saw only the sea below and a smudge on the eastern horizon that must be Florida.

The pilot was very good at his job, and put them down on the runway without a bump. Carras saw the thrust reverser pop up on the wing and then they were easing to a stop. Isaac came through the lounge to the rear door and had it open before Carras and Hilary were out of their plush seats. Two men in olive work clothes pushed a set of stairs into position and Hilary and Carras followed Isaac out into the outside heat. Carras took off his suit jacket and undid his tie, blinking at the change in the intensity of light, looking around.

The runway arrowed off into the distance and was lost in heat haze. In the other direction, Carras expected to see some kind of airport and realized he hadn't brought his passport. But there was only a hangar and a blacktopped road that went off in the direction of the hill and was soon lost beneath the riot of tropical greenery that surrounded the airstrip. Private island, he thought.

"Where are we?" he wanted to know.

"Not yet," she said. "Trust me. Please."

He shrugged and spread his hands, then said, "Is all this yours?"

She made a little sound in the back of her throat, and said, "No."

Isaac had gone into the hangar. Now he came out at the wheel of a Range Rover, stopped beside them and got out. "Doctor," he said, "my employer has asked me to give you a tour of the island and answer any questions, except two—who he is and why he wants to talk to you. He wants to do that himself."

Now the light didn't seem quite so bright. Carras turned to Hilary. "So I'm not your guest," he said.

"It'll be all right," she said.

"Doctor," Isaac said, "my employer likes to do things his own way, but he means you no harm. On the contrary."

Carras half expected to see Leonard Maigrot step out of the bushes, like Rod Serling in an old *Twilight Zone* episode, though he couldn't believe that Hilary Cartiere would be involved in anything sinister. But to be sure, he said to Isaac, "Can I get on that jet and go back to Miami right now?"

"Yes, sir."

"Okay then, that's what I want to do."

He turned and walked back to the jet, began to climb the stairs. He heard Hilary call his name then the sound of her footsteps on the tarmac, but he didn't look back and kept going until he was back in the aircraft's lounge. Hilary's expression was hard to read.

Isaac followed them and said, "I'll go speak to the crew. They'll have to file an amended flight plan, but we should be airborne in a couple of minutes."

He went to the door leading forward. It opened and the young blonde poked her head out, looking confused.

"Wait," Carras said.

Isaac turned. "Yes, sir?"

"It's all right. I'll stay."

"Yes, sir."

"I just wanted to be sure I could leave whenever I wanted."

Hilary looked at him as if he'd just told a lame joke. "Of course, you can," she said.

They went back out onto the tarmac. Carras took out his cell phone and checked its display. It said he was still connected to the world. "Okay," he said, and smiled at Hilary. "We'll call it an unexpected vacation. I'd done everything I wanted to do at the conference anyway."

She smiled back, full power, and said, "Let's get going."

Isaac opened the rear door of the Range Rover and they got in. They turned onto a road that paralleled the island's shore. Carras thought the route was much wider than the amount of traffic on one small island could justify. He noticed, too, that when they came to a curve, the road widened even more and banked sharply upwards.

"Are we on some kind of race track?" he asked.

Isaac answered from the front seat. "My employer's son is a racing driver, sir. It's his practice track."

The information confirmed for Carras that the island belonged to Terry Flynnt. He realized that the knowledge ought to have diminished some of the magic that surrounded his until-now miraculous encounter with the movie star. But it didn't. If Flynnt was willing to go to these lengths just to get Carras to listen to an offer, he probably deserved to be listened to. Besides, Carras could admit to himself that Flynnt's penchant for mystery was not much to put up with as the price for a day in paradise with Hilary Cartiere.

Hilary said to Isaac, "Is there a good place to swim here?" She put her hand on Carras's arm, and he felt the warmth through his shirt sleeve. "Would you like to take a swim, Athan?"

"I don't have a suit."

"I don't think we'll need them," she said. "Will we, Isaac?"

"The island is completely private," he said. "No one will bother you."

She squeezed Carras's arm. "This looks like it," she said.

The Range Rover came around a curve and he saw a building that might have been airlifted whole from the French Riviera: solid white walls, red tiled roof, a stone flagged patio and black iron grillwork climbed by sturdy vines that produced bright colored blossoms Carras couldn't name. Isaac stopped the vehicle and let them out.

"I think you'll find everything you need inside, but if not just pick up the phone," he said. "The main house is up the hill. Somebody will bring you lunch. In the meantime, the beach shelves very gradually and the water is clear."

"Let's get some towels," Hilary said and went into the villa.

Carras said, "When do I meet the mystery man?"

"Tomorrow, sir," Isaac said. "He's not on the island at the moment."

"All right," Carras said. "I'll play along."

"Let me know if there's anything you need."

Hilary came back outside carrying beach towels, a basket and a large folded umbrella. "I think I have everything I need," Carras said.

The sand began only a few feet from the villa's door, white and fine as powder. They set up the umbrella and laid out the towels. The basket held a selection of bottled beer, wine and fruit juices. "I found them in the refrigerator," Hilary said.

She was wearing a simple sleeveless dress and sandals. Now she kicked off the latter and pulled the former over her head. She wore no bra, nor did she need one: her breasts were still full and upturned as they had been in *Five Bullets*. Carras's surgeon's eye would have detected the work of a plastic surgeon. He saw no sign of it. Though she must be well past forty, Hilary Cartiere was pure perfection.

She said, "Yes, they are nice, aren't they?" He was embarrassed to be caught staring, but when she gently lifted her breasts in her hands, he couldn't look away.

"Get your things off," she said. "I'm getting in that water." She turned her back on him and slid her panties down to her ankles, showing him yet more perfection, then ran down the beach and into the gentle surf. She walked out a few yards then dove into the blue.

Carras tore off his clothes and pulled off his shoes and socks. The sun's full force struck his skin like heat from an open oven, but the breeze from the sea lifted the hairs on his limbs and cooled his torso. He saw Hilary swimming with a strong stroke out to where it was deeper.

He knew he had been manipulated to bring him to this place and time, knew he ought to be thinking about the situation he had walked into, weighing the uncertainties that surrounded him like a careful physician, but the sight of Hilary Cartiere as he had always desired to see her had brought him fully erect and right now he preferred to think like a surgeon. He walked into the water, cut its surface with a clean, swift dive and swam straight toward her.

Chapter 6

When his mother called upstairs to let him know that breakfast was ready, Costas shouted back, "A minute!" without looking up from the workbench he had built across one corner of his room. He delicately laid the end of the thin silver wire on the terminal and touched the tip of the soldering iron to it. Three more touches and the circuit was made. He slipped the two little nickel-cadmium batteries into their holders, and the machine was ready go.

Costas rubbed the back of his neck and regarded his creation. It was not an impressive sight: a two-square inch piece of plastic circuit board with a computer chip and the watch battery power source on top and two rows of tiny electric motors connected to miniature wheels underneath. A simple ligh-sensitive cell sat on the front of the device.

"Come on, the pancakes are going cold!" his mother's voice called.

"Just a second!" Costas set the little machine at the base of a simple tee-maze he had made in a cardboard box and positioned a small reading light to shine on one end of the crossbar. He flicked the microswitch that started the device and waited until he saw it begin to creep forward. There would be nothing to see until it had made its laborious way to the end of the maze. He went downstairs to eat.

He gave the cooled pancakes a thirty seconds-long microwave bath, then joined his mother at the table by the window that overlooked the merlot vines.

"I'm testing it now," he said, before forking a wad of pancake and blueberry syrup into his mouth.

"I hope it works," Beth said.

His mouth too full to talk, he made a *me too* face.

"We need to talk about this trip with your father," she said.

Costas felt his features alter their arrangement, knew that it was an automatic response so ingrained in him that he could observe it as if it were happening to somebody else.

"Don't do that," his mother said and he nodded and began to chew again.

Nothing was said for a long moment, then Costas swallowed and took a sip of his orange juice. His mouth still felt dry. "I don't want to do this," he said.

"You have to."

"Why? I've got along all right without him till now."

His mother put her hand on his arm. "No," she said, "you haven't."

He cut another wedge of pancake and paused with the fork almost to his mouth. The motion made his mother's hand fall away. "I'm okay," he said.

"No. You're not."

He chewed and swallowed. "Why? Cause I didn't remember the dumb car? I was just a little kid."

"You were ten, and you loved that car. When your dad took you out in it your eyes were like Christmas morning." She looked out at the sunny hillside with the vines on their supports but Costas knew she was seeing another place and time. "You never called it 'the car'—always 'the Pantera,'" she said. "It was, 'Dad, can we take the Pantera out on Saturday?' or 'Dad, do you want to wash the Pantera?'"

"So, okay, I had a thing about the car. Lots of little kids are car crazy. So what?"

"So how could you forget about it, and I mean completely?" Beth said. "When you saw that Pantera down at the mall, why didn't you say, 'Gee, my father had one of those when I was a kid?'"

"I've been busy," Costas said. "It slipped my mind."

"Ha ha," Beth said, deadpan. But then her face softened. "Costas, I know it hurt, I know it still hurts, but you can't cut yourself off from your whole childhood, just because one bad thing—even one really bad thing—happened to you."

"How does riding in a car make nine years not happen?"

"It doesn't. But you have to get over it some time."

"Why?"

"Because you're not going to know who you are until you know your father."

Costas said nothing, chewed more pancake and drank more juice. But in the end he couldn't resist asking the question. "Why not? What is he to me?"

Beth made a *What can I tell you?* face and said, "That's up to you to decide. But I can tell you, sitting here across the table from you, it's like I'm looking at a home video of your father when we met."

Costas pushed away the empty plate and stood up. "I got to go see how my experiment is coming."

Beth let him go without commenting that he not only looked just like his father but said exactly the same things.

When Costas got back to his room, the little machine had crawled all the way to the end of the maze. He lifted it out and put it on the work bench and reached for the octopus of wires coming from his oscilloscope. He tested the circuit that led from the controlling chip to the wheel motors on one side, then tested the matching circuit on the other. He noted down the readings then rechecked them. The figures didn't alter on the second check.

"Holy shit," he said. "It works."

The neural network had worked. The inanimate transistors and resistors had come to life. They had learned the pattern and, they had anticipated the path and they had performed, knowing that the rewarded behavior would be to turn toward the light.

"The Costas Circuit," he chuckled. Enough of these little babies wired together and you could make a pretty smart machine. Costas started up at the ceiling. Wow. Imagine a billion of them on a chip.

The young man let out a little sound. He had done it. He had built the simplest possible equivalent of a brain *circuit*, an electronic network that got more efficient the more it was used. It was the electro-chemical equivalent of how the brain learned by doing.

"Wait until they see this," he said.

"What?" said his mother, and he turned to see her standing in the doorway.

He smiled and said, "Well, don't tell anybody, but I think your son has just invented one of the key components of artificial intelligence."

She came over and stood behind him, put her hands on his shoulders. "Your father will be very proud of you," she said.

Costas looked back at the little machine. "We'll see," he said.

• • •

Carras and Hilary swam together in water that was almost as clear as air. They dove to the bottom, finding shells and little many-legged things that scuttled out of their way or dug themselves into the sand. Each time he reached for her she rolled and flipped and scooted away—but never too far away, and not before allowing his hand to linger a moment on a breast or thigh.

Finally, she stopped and stood where the water was waist deep. He came to her and put his arms around her, cupped her perfect buttocks and pulled her close, his rigid penis trapped between their bellies. She smiled at him and slid a hand in from his thigh to cup his testicles and gently squeeze. He couldn't keep the moan from escaping.

"Let's go inside," she said. She took him by the hand and they came out of the sea, scooped up the towels and dried themselves as they walked through a clutch of palm trees to the villa.

It was shady under the palms but the villa's walls caught the glare from the sea and the bright sand and shed a dull glow through the gloom. Inside, the rooms were high-ceilinged and plastered in creamy white, the floors red-tiled with a few patterned rugs. The furniture was dark wood and stuffed leather and the art on the walls looked to have been chosen for starkness of line and color.

But Carras saw nothing but Hilary toweling herself dry, standing with her legs apart so that he could see the pink line of her sex through the reddish gold hairs that were beaded with droplets of the sea between her legs.

His groin ached now and a droplet of his own glistened at the end of it. He went to her, but she held him gently at a distance and said, "Let me do this the way I planned, so it will be perfect for you."

"You're perfect for me," he said, but he let her lead him to the couch. He sat, although his erect member remained standing, and she bent to stroke it from scrotum to tip, saying, "Not long now."

She went into the bedroom and came back with a small flat box. Carras thought, *Oh god, not drugs*, but his moment of despair vanished when she went to a freestanding cupboard that faced the couch on the other side of the room and opened the doors. Inside was a wide-screen digital TV with a DVD player and now he saw that the box in her hand contained a disk.

"It's The Cut," she said. "The studio had it remastered but the DVD hasn't been released yet."

It was his favorite of all her movies. She played an OR nurse and Harrison Ford was a surgeon, both of them married to different people, but they fall for each other. When the doctor's wife disappears, suspicion falls on the adulterous pair. The plot was standard potboiler, but Hilary was good—Carras thought it a career-best performance—playing a strong woman made vulnerable by her own passion. There had been an Academy Award nomination. Carras had seen it on the big screen twice when it was first out, once more at university film club screening, and several times on video.

The DVD version was miraculous, recapturing as video never could the luminous quality that made Hilary Cartiere one of the outstanding faces in film. "Hank Hitchens lit me," she said, sitting beside him on the couch as the first scene came up. "He was wonderful."

"You were the one who was wonderful," Carras said. He put his arm around her shoulders and she guided his hand to her breast. He turned toward her, hungry, but she said, "Watch," and turned his head back toward the screen, her fingertips gently firm on his jaw.

The film opened in an operating room, the doctor and nurse communicating professionally by their voices, but sending a different message through their eyes. Then came a dissolve to a motel cabin by a lake, two cars outside, and a tracking shot into the window of the little room. A thin bar of sunlight across a bed, two naked lovers seen only in a shifting montage of body parts, the camera swooping in and gliding out, and over it all the voices of Harrison Ford and Hilary Cartiere.

"I wish it could be like this forever," said the digitally rendered voice from the speakers. "Just us, like this. Nobody else."

As he heard the familiar lines, Carras felt the soft puff of her breath on his cheek and realized that she was speaking the words into his ear.

Harrison Ford said something, then Hilary's voice came low and rich. "We could find a place somewhere, let it all go."

On the screen, her face lay on the actor's bare stomach, then slid down and out of shot. And now Hilary was slipping to the floor to kneel between his legs.

"This is..." Carras wanted to say "heaven" but before he could find the word she had him in her mouth, her fingers languidly stroking the shaft. A sound of helplessness came out of him.

The scene rolled on. Now it was Hilary on her back, the sun glowing in her cheekbones, her mouth open as her arousal swept her toward completion. Carras looked from one Hilary to another while the sensations created by her swirling, flickering tongue and pressing lips pulled him into her wondrous mouth. Then, as the Hilary of the motel room made a broken gasp of pleasure, her fingers slid past the sac of his balls and lightly touched the sensitive flesh beyond, a feathery tickle that had him instantly spurting into her, the orgasm searing his cock like hot wires, while she sucked and squeezed and swallowed until he was limp and drained.

"Why can't it always be like this?" the Hilary on the screen whispered.

• • •

It was hours later. They were in the bedroom, the sheets of the oversized bed swirled and tumbled under and over them. They had made love then lunch had arrived. They ate, came back to the bedroom, did it again then slept. Now they lay awake on their backs, fingers entwined.

"We have to talk," Carras said. A part of him said, *Don't do this, just enjoy the moment,* but a stronger voice said, *things have to be said.* He rolled on his side to face her and said, "I know about Terry Flynnt."

She said nothing, stared at the ceiling.

"Is he a friend of yours?" he asked.

She turned her face to him now. "I met him for the first time a few days ago."

"Our meeting at the hotel, that was no accident."

"No, no accident." She looked at him, her perfect upper teeth biting gently at her full lower lip, and waited for him to go on. When he didn't, she said, "How did you know it was Flynnt? He was very clear that I wasn't to tell you."

"His guy, Maigrot is his name..."

"He's the one who first contacted me."

"Same here," Carras said. "I asked around. The size of the jet and the race track pretty well clinched it."

She nodded. "Are you mad at me for getting you here?"

Carras shook his head. "No, never. Whatever Flynnt has in mind, he's given me the most wonderful day I've had in longer than I can remember. Being here with you is like a Hollywood blockbuster—compared to which, my regular life is a re-run of a black-and-white situation comedy from the fifties."

She rolled toward him, put an arm across his chest. He felt her breasts nudging his side. "Mmm," she said. "I always like a good review."

"There's just one thing."

"What?"

"Flynnt didn't pressure you to do this, did he? He didn't threaten you or anything?"

"No," she said. "No pressure, no threats."

"'Cause if he did, I'll clean his clock."

She stroked his chest. "You're sweet."

"But I'd like to know..."

She waited, then said, "What?"

Let it go, said the voice in Carras's head, but he had to ask. "Why did you do this? Did he pay you?"

She was very still. "I'm not a whore," she said.

"I didn't..." he began.

"Yes, I was hired to bring you here." She raised herself up on one elbow. "You want to know the price? A picture. Guaranteed financing, I pick the director and I get script approval. Athan, I would do a lot for that kind of deal,

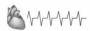

but I wouldn't do just anything. Or with just anyone."

"I wanted you to see this from my point of view," he said. "It's like I walked into a dream. The idea that it might be only a dream—worse, that it might be Flynnt using my dream to get something from me—well, that would be hard to take."

She said, "Okay, now I want you see it from my side. When he asked me to do this, I said, 'Who is he, this doctor?' They gave me a big file on you, newspaper clippings, articles you'd written, that piece in *People* magazine and the awful things they wrote about you when that other doctor died. I saw videos of you speaking at conferences and all the TV interviews. I saw this honest, sincere man who saves people's lives and who got a really raw deal he didn't deserve."

She touched her fingertips to his cheek. "Do you know how many people like you I get to meet? None. I meet producers and directors and agents who are so full of shit they have to hire people to shovel it for them. I meet actors who think the sun shines out of their surgically altered butts but at the same time they're terrified one day the phone's going to stop ringing because that's the day they will no longer be able to get a good table at Spago's and then they might as well truck on back to Cow Dump, Arkansas.

"I get to meet reporters who say, 'Hey didn't you used to be Hilary Cartiere?' and I meet one hell of a lot of men who want to fuck me because when they were fifteen they had that poster—the one with the see-through shirt?—on the ceiling over their bed."

She moved her hands down to his waist then joined them at the small of his back and put her cheek on his chest. "So when I get to meet a decent guy who still thinks I'm twenty-three, a guy who actually does some good in the world, I say, 'All right, let's meet this guy and see what happens.' So here I am."

"I'm sorry," he said.

She looked down at him then bent her head and kissed him softly on the lips. "No," she said, "in a world full of sorry-ass bastards, you're one of the few good ones."

He reached for her and realized he was hard again. *Just like when I was fifteen and had that poster on the wall*, he thought. *His mother wouldn't allow it on the ceiling.*

It was another hour before they came out of the bedroom to find that someone had laid out a mini-buffet, complete with heated chafing dishes, in the dining room. After they ate, they watched *The Cut* again, then took a walk along the beach.

"This has been the best day of my life," he told her.

"Same here," she said. She lifted her lips to be kissed, her eyes closed. *She couldn't help acting*, he thought. *You are what you do.*

The moon had risen, only half full, and was casting a steel-gray light on the ocean. A surprisingly cool breeze came off the water as Carras went down to where the waves were rippling up the beach. The only sound was the hiss of bursting bubbles in the sea foam.

They walked back toward the villa. After a while, Carras said, "What can you tell me about Terry Flynnt?"

"I only met him the one time."

"What did you think of him?"

She shrugged. "Everybody thinks that the power people in Hollywood are the big name producers and directors. But the real power is in the money, and that belongs to the people who run the corporations who own the studios." She stopped and looked at the moon on the water. "I've met some of them, and Flynnt is the same kind. He's used to getting what he wants. No question he's hard. I'm sure he could be cruel. I'd be careful about crossing him. Very careful."

Her hand was warm in his. He wondered what tomorrow would bring. Clearly, Flynnt was courting him. The only thing that Carras could imagine would have caught the billionaire's interest was his research. You didn't have to hire movie stars to consult a heart surgeon.

So there would be an offer, and it would have something to do with his research. Maybe a big grant. It struck him all at once that Flynnt must have been the power from on high who had cooled his chances with the Fallon Foundation. Flynnt would have wanted any complications cleared out of the way before making his own bid. That should have made him mad, he thought, but he had to admit he was more curious than angry. He couldn't really complain about how the day had ended up.

Carras was sure the offer would be worth thinking about. There would probably be money on the table, more than he had ever made as an academic. But the money was not a major temptation, not compared to the freedom to pursue his research. And if the relationship he thought was developing with Hilary continued, he could be a man who was literally living his dreams.

He let himself think about it, imagining what it would be like to leave teaching and surgery, to run a first-class research outfit, to develop techniques that would revolutionize medical science. And to come home to Hilary Cartiere, who was everything he'd ever wanted her to be and more. It was a big-budget, technicolor dream life, compared to which the way he had lived the past several years was a monochrome B-movie.

Of course, she'd probably need to spend some time in Hollywood. Her work was important to her. But they could have one of those long-distance relationships—his schedule would be whatever he wanted it to be, and how many pictures a year could she want to do?

He let the cool water wash over his feet, soaking the cuffs of his new pants.

A shiver went up his spine. He looked at the moon's reflection in the calm sea and thought, I could get used to this. *Hell, I deserve this. I've done more than most people could do in ten lifetimes.* He had saved enough lives to fill an old-fashioned movie palace.

I'll listen to what the man has to say, he thought. *And if the offer's good, I'll take it.*

• • •

Carras woke early. Hilary lay wrapped in the covers, gently snoring. A warm scent of woman came from her when he leaned over and softly kissed the hair above her temple. He looked at her and saw that, sleeping, her face was subtly different from her waking image. There was a little more looseness to her flesh, as if the waking Hilary Cartiere maintained a firmness of jaw line by conscious will.

He got out of bed and used the bathroom, then went through into the villa's sitting room, intending to walk down to the sea and swim. He always liked a vigorous workout before breakfast if he could get it, especially when he was facing any kind of test—and he was sure that today's meeting with Terry Flynnt would test him in some way.

He didn't get to the beach. When he opened the door he saw a racing bicycle leaning against a palm tree in front of the villa. Arrayed neatly on the ground beside it were a pair of cycling shorts, a tank top, a pair of sneakers and a helmet.

At first he thought they had brought his own machine from the storage lockers in the basement of his Yale apartment block. It was the same model, a Cannondale R5000 Si in Saeco Team racing colors, with a sixth-generation advanced aluminum design frame hand-crafted at the maker's Bedford, Connecticut workshop. It had the same Slice Si fork and the Hollowgram crank and bottom bracket which cut a full pound off the bike's weight. The combined shift and brake levers were from Ergopower and the feather-light wheels and hubs were Campagnolo Nucleons. It was a sixteen pound, two-wheeled rocket, and like the Pantera, it was a perfect marriage of American and Italian engineering styles.

It was exactly the bicycle that Carras had put together for himself, with the aid and advice of New Haven's best bike shop. He could tell just by looking that the adjustments of seat, handle bars and brakes would be perfect for his frame. When he pulled it away from the tree and gave it a closer examination, he half expected to see the engraving of his Social Security number on the frame's underside, so he could identify it if it were stolen, but the paint was unmarked.

Flynnt's people had gone to the trouble of exactly recreating Carras's own bike, then left it casually leaning against the nearest tree so that he could indulge himself in a morning ride. Which was exactly what anyone who knew him well would expect him to feel like doing after waking up in paradise next to a woman he had wanted all his life. The trouble was, these people who knew him so precisely were complete strangers to him. They weren't friends who had honestly come by a close familiarity with the ins and outs of Athan Carras. He imagined them as a horde of faceless functionaries in lab coats, equipped with calculators and measuring tapes, hovering in the background of his life and trying to learn everything about him. He wondered what, if anything, they had missed.

He went inside, changed into the cycling gear and filled the bike's water bottle. A minute later, he wheeled from the villa's access road onto the island-circling race track and began to climb the bike's impeccably tuned gears. The machine was smooth and, as he had guessed, in perfect proportion to his length of leg and arm. He dug in and the bike went away with him as if some invisible force was pulling him down the track.

The sea was on his right, the sun only just clearing the horizon. The air was clear and still cool from the night. Carras breathed deeply and upped his pace, curling over the handlebars, the wind tugging at his cheeks. The track was mostly flat, but some of the curves climbed a little, following the contours of the ground. Carras swept up the inclines as if they weren't there, leaned in at a steep angle as he took the curves.

He hadn't ridden in a place like this in a long time: no traffic, no stop signs or merging lanes, no skate boarders hot-dogging on narrow asphalt paths that were supposed to be for cyclists only. This was pure biking, a simplicity of motion and forward movement, lacking only the participation of another human being on another perfect piece of machinery—to make the ride a race.

Carras came to the top of an ascending curve and straightened up in the seat to look back the way he had come. He could see almost a mile before greenery got in the way, and at the limit of his vision he saw a flash of sunlight on polished metal. When the dazzle ended, he saw motion. Another cyclist was on the track, and moving fast toward him.

All right, Carras thought. *Let's see what you've got. Bring it on.*

He dug in, steadily ratcheting up his pace until he was leaning over the handlebars, letting the streamlined helmet cut the wind and slip it around his body. He felt the big quad muscles in his thighs begin to hum, the femoral biceps on the backs of his legs stretching further as each heel came down to the lowest part of its pedal's rotation. When the muscles settled into the rhythm, he upped the pace again, then repeated the process. The asphalt fled beneath him like a gray river at full flood, and the whir of the tires against the smooth surface mixed with the rush of wind flying past his ears.

He had lost track of time now, couldn't have said whether it was five minutes or ten since he had seen the flash of light from behind him. There was another slope coming up and he decided he would sit upright at its top and look back to see how his competitor was doing. He was sure he had put more distance between them. He put his head down and increased the effort, buying himself the seconds he would waste in the backward glance.

There was a flicker of motion in the peripheral range of his left eye. Carras inclined his head a little to bring whatever had caught his attention into focus, and saw a black shape, a shadow, on the hurtling ground beside him. The rising sun was now at his back, the road having curved toward the west a mile or two back, and the shadow was elongated past the point of any recognizability. What was clear, though, was that it was gaining on him—had already, just in the time he had been looking at it, come level with his handlebars and was moving past his wheel.

Carras grunted and increased his speed, seeing the edge of the shadow fall back and become lost behind him. He set a speed that was almost a sprint, a speed he could not hold for long on rising ground. But he reasoned that whoever was coming up behind him must have been burning energy at just such a high rate of expenditure and would soon tire.

The warm hum of effort in his thighs was becoming the painful heat of burn-out. The muscle cells were consuming their supplies of energy-giving sugar and filling with a residue of lactic acid. But Carras pushed harder. Another thirty seconds to the top of the slope, then ease back, he told himself. Yet even as he heard the words in his head, he saw the shadow reappear at the edge of his vision and steadily move forward.

Push it! said the voice in his head. *Come on!* He could feel the long muscles of his thighs trembling with strain, his bunched calves wanting to cramp with each contraction. His mouth was open now, his diaphragm gulping breath into his lungs as he made the top of the grade and looked for a down slope that would let him slacken enough to ease the pain in his legs. But there was no descent. The road continued level for a couple of hundred yards before climbing again.

He wasn't more than halfway along the brief flat before the shadow caught him and moved past again. When he reached the bottom of the next incline the leading edge of the shadow was ahead of his front wheel, and as he dug in again it continued to move past him. He set the best pace he could without throwing away every ounce of his reserves, thinking, *he's got to be tiring too,* but the shadow flowed past him like an inevitability.

This slope was longer and steeper than the last one, and before he had climbed more than a third of it the shadow beside him was replaced by a more solid presence: first a hissing wheel, then a pair of tanned legs pumping steadily at racing speed, then another wheel, then too soon the nothing of empty pavement.

Now Carras pulled the last shreds of strength out of legs that were shivering and screaming in pain, demanded that burning lungs pull another increment of fuel from the morning air. He would pull level and pass the other rider, just one time. That would be enough. It would salve his ego. Then he would stop, offer to call it a draw and take the measure of whoever had given him such a run for his money. He flashed on a memory of Cory Goldenberg's assessment of him, that he hated to lose. Well, he could accept a draw with honor.

He expected his opponent would be some twenty-something hard body with nothing better to do than train for hours every day, a ringer that Flynnt had sicced on Carras just to unsettle him before they opened negotiations on whatever the billionaire wanted. He'd read that big business types played such mind games with each other.

But though he strained beyond what he had always thought were his limits, until his thighs trembled like an old wino after a dry night, the other rider's rear wheel never appeared in the topmost edge of his downward focused vision. He reached the top of the hill with lungs that felt seared and with acid bile creeping up his throat, and looked ahead to where a man in shorts and singlet stood leaning against what looked to be an identical bike to his own, a few dozen yards along the now level road. He wasn't even breathing hard.

Carras stopped and set a foot down on the asphalt, letting the air flow in and out of his open mouth until his breathing was under control and his legs no longer felt that they were made of some thin liquid barely contained by skin. Then he walked the bike forward until he was level with the other man.

"I'm Terry Flynnt," the man said.

Carras knew his face was betraying his surprise, knew it from the gotcha! look that briefly registered in the other man's expression. Flynnt took off his helmet to reveal sandy hair with only a light frosting of gray. The eyes were a pale blue, the color of ancient ice. The features could have been planed and carved from some rare and tightly grained hardwood, a face that looked to have been scraped down to its essentials. The voice that came out of the hard-lipped mouth was used to telling others how it was going to be.

Carras made an effort to recover his poise. "I hear you want to make me some kind of offer," he said.

He had been wondering what kind of man Flynnt would turn out to be, once he emerged from the shadows. He hadn't expected to feel warm and friendly to a man who was so partial to manipulating others. But he also hadn't expected to dislike the man on sight.

It was a rare reaction for Carras. The strength of it surprised him. He couldn't recall ever disliking anyone on sight. He remembered again what Goldenberg had said, but he rejected the notion that his aversion to the other man originated from being beaten in a race. There was something else about Flynnt. Carras sensed that here was a man dedicated to denying the common mystery, a man who intended to make himself rigid and smooth all the way to the core.

Now Carras found himself being looked over, the other man's eyes running over him like a horse buyer at a stockyard sale. Still Flynnt said nothing, and Carras came to a conclusion that he didn't expect to alter: he did not want to work for this man. *He's got way too high an opinion of himself,* he thought.

After a leisurely inspection, Flynnt nodded to himself and said, "I want to show you something." He raised his hand and Carras heard the sound of a vehicle's engine revving to climb the hill that had just defeated him. The Range Rover appeared with Isaac at the wheel.

"We'll leave the bikes," Flynnt said, letting his bicycle fall and tossing his helmet after it. Carras did the same, though he lowered his bike carefully to the pavement. He could hear his father: it was a sin to damage a well made machine.

The driver held the rear door for them and they got in. "Where are we going?" Carras said, but Flynnt's lean, spidery-fingered hand just waved the question away. The answer came soon enough.

The Range Rover followed the track down toward the beach and through the trees on the landward side Carras saw concrete and glass. They turned into a driveway that ended at a four-story building. Isaac parked before the main doors.

Inside the building was cool and silent, the only sound the waft of the air conditioning system. There was a foyer on the other side of which were two large double doors, and behind them was a corridor with more doors that opened on rooms that had laboratory benches with sinks in them, equipment racks and steel cupboards, desks with computers and printers. There was a conference room and a cafeteria and a concrete-floored space fitted out with pens and cages. Carras wondered if Hilary's joke about Dr. Moreau was closer to the mark than she'd meant it to be.

"Obviously, this is a research facility," he said. "What kind of research are you doing here?"

Again, Flynnt waved away the question. "Upstairs," he said. An elevator took them up one floor. Here the building was an apartment block, with small, one and two bedroom units, with furnishings and appliances of good quality. They looked into a couple of the apartments, then went up another floor. Here the units were fewer but larger, the furnishings better than merely good, with views over the trees of the sea and the hill that dominated the north end of the island.

Then they went to the top floor. The elevator opened on one vast penthouse apartment, opulently fitted and furnished, its seaside wall an unbroken expanse of glass. Carras went across the deep piled carpet to the wall of glass, until his view was filled by the sea.

He had always liked the sea, liked the idea of it. Maybe it was some gene passed down from his ancestors, all those ancient Greeks with their boats pulled up on shore, sitting around a fire and talking about what was over the horizon or under the waves. He watched the breakers come in and thought, *This is a mind-clearing view. This is the kind of place where a man could get above it all and think.*

The master bedroom alone was larger than Carras's entire apartment in the Yale campus housing, the bed big enough for a demi-god. The en suite bathroom was the size of a seminar room, its jacuzzi like something from an Italian science fiction movie.

They went back to the main room with its sweep of sea and sky. "What do you think?" Flynnt said.

Carras used the only word he could think of. "I'm flabbergasted. Is this where you live?"

Flynnt looked like the kind of man who had forgotten how to be amused, but now a faint memory of a smile touched his lips. "No," he said, "this is where you live. All of this is for you—and a lot more."

Chapter 7

Carras had spent his professional career among people who brimmed with self-assurance. Cardiothoracic surgery was not a business for self-doubters; the opening up of human beings and replacement of their living hearts called for a degree of nerve that was not often found outside the ranks of test pilots and matadors.

But Terry Flynnt's bald statement—this is where you will live—conveyed to Carras a certainty even beyond the sense of assurance that was to be expected among the very rich. There should have been an "if" after that declaration—this is where you will live if you accept my offer.

The building they were in was new and unused. The labs had none of the umistakeable odors that accumulate from biomedical research. The residential areas had no lived-in look. "This is a brand new facility," he said. "You went ahead and built this for me?"

Carras thought he'd put a good dose of skepticism into the tone of his question, but it didn't seem to register on Terry Flynnt.

"There's more," the billionaire said. "It's a package offer. You get the research facility, which is yours to do with as you see fit. Plus a budget sufficient to hire any staff you need, at salaries competitive with other institutions."

He was ticking the points off on his fingers. "For yourself, a salary commensurate with your stature in the research community. Shall we say triple what you're making now, plus a generous living allowance?"

A fourth finger down. "And an endowment fund of one billion dollars, the interest from which you can disburse to other researchers in whatever way you see fit."

Carras wished he'd saved the word flabbergasted for how he felt now. Flynnt had just made him the most amazing offer in the history of medical research. Hell, Carras thought, the research facility and a fat salary in paradise were astonishing all on their own. But the endowment fund! Carras didn't know how much a billion dollars could be made to safely yield, year after year, but it could easily be a hundred million. Skillfully invested, it might be double that.

With command of his own institute plus a hundred million or two to dole out to other scientists every year, he would instantly rocket to the highest ranks of the research establishment. He would wield incredible power. Having just had the experience of asking for but not receiving a DHCA research grant that was by comparison a pittance, he was now being offered the equivalent of a promotion from pilgrim to pope.

The religious comparison snapped him back into focus. Flynnt had played him effortlessly, got him thinking about the reward before he had vouchsafed word one about what must be done to earn it—just like the devil in one of the old tales.

The man was looking at him now, the hard blue eyes unblinking, waiting for a response. *Something is wrong here*, Carras thought. Nobody would go to all this trouble unless there was something—he heard Charlie Vance's voice saying *hinky* in the back of his head—and thought, *yeah, there's something hinky about this.*

There was more than self-confidence in Flynnt's attitude, more than the assurance of a rich man indulging himself. Carras sensed something behind the too-still face, the too-controlled voice, a raw emotion ruthlessly concealed—desperation, maybe, or the fierce intensity of a fanatic. Whatever it was, something told him to back away.

"It's an amazing offer, Mr. Flynnt, but I'm going to have to turn it down."

Flynnt's face didn't change, but the intensity of his stare somehow seemed to deepen. Still, his voice was without emotion. "Why?"

The pieces were now falling into place for Athan Carras. "Because I think I know what you want me to do for you. And it's impossible—not to mention grossly unethical."

Flynnt's eyebrows rose minimally. "And just what do you think I want you to do for me?"

"Well, it's obvious, isn't it?" Carras said.

They might have been discussing the time of day for all the feeling that was in the billionaire's voice. "Is it?"

"You've done a hell of a background check on me, so you know about my research into deep hypothermic cardiac arrest. The way I see it, you got interested in me because you came across the paper I published on the preliminary experiments into DHCA. You learned that I was applying for a grant to take that research to the next level, so you used your power to block the Fallon Foundation grant so that you could offer to fund me instead. Fund me and control me."

He stopped, and waited for Flynnt to react but all the man said was, "Please continue."

"You're aging," Carras went on. "You've got wealth and power, and you don't want to give them up. I just have to look at you to see that you've been driving yourself to an absurd level of fitness for your age. Why else would you do that except to try to lengthen your lifespan? But you also know that you've got maybe a dozen more years before no amount of effort will hold off the inevitable."

Again, Carras paused but again there was no response, except, "This is fascinating, doctor. Let me hear it all."

Carras was beginning to feel foolish. The man played games, he thought, like the business with the bike race, and every game must be a zero-sum contest, producing a winner and a loser, and the winner always had to be Terry Flynnt.

"All right," he said. "You figure that maybe twenty years from now the current research into the human genome and stem cells will bring about true regeneration therapies. Those who can afford them might live to be a hundred and thirty or forty years old, enjoying active, productive lives. But you can't wait another twenty years; you might be too far gone by then. You might get a longer life, but it would be just a longer decline.

"So you're hoping that I can put you into cold sleep for those twenty years, let you wake up in time to lay your hands on another fifty years or more of being rich and powerful." Carras shrugged. "But it's a layman's fantasy. Science fiction. I can't do it. And I wouldn't even try, because it would require experimenting on you—and I've already said that would be grossly unethical."

Even with Flynnt's consent, Carras could not place the man under DHCA. The technique was still in its developmental infancy. There was no guarantee—there were not even good odds—that after twenty years in suspended animation Terry Flynnt could be brought back to life. Even if his heart and lungs could be restarted, his brain might easily have deteriorated to the point where he became permanently comatose—a vegetable.

The Hippocratic oath's first requirement was that a doctor do no harm.

Putting Terry Flynnt into cold sleep, willing though he might be, would violate that oath. Carras would not do it.

Carras thought he detected the faintest of smiles playing around Flynnt's mouth. He had the feeling he was wasting his reason on a man whose mind was made up, and who was determined to have his way.

"So you've gone to a lot of trouble for nothing," he said. "I'll always be grateful that you made it possible for me to meet Hilary Cartiere, but I think all of this expense could have been avoided if your man Maigrot had told me what you were after."

The smile on Flynnt's face was definite now. "So that's what you think, is it?"

Both the expression and tone bespoke amusement. Again, Carras felt that he had been wrong-footed to put him at a disadvantage.

"I don't care for games, Mr. Flynnt," he said. "I want to leave now."

The amusement fled from the billionaire's face. *He's not used to people talking to him like that*, Carras thought. *Well, tough shit.*

Flynnt said, "I couldn't care less about your research, doctor. You can do whatever the hell you want with this facility, but I can assure you I won't be part of your experiments."

Again, Carras felt like he'd been made to look right by an opponent who was going left. "Then what the hell do you want from me?"

"You're a heart surgeon," Flynnt said. "What do you think I'm after?"

"There's nothing wrong with your heart," Carras said. "You more than proved that on the bike."

"I'm not the patient. Come with me." Again the slight smile. "Unless you want to leave without knowing what this is really all about."

The Range Rover took them along the track to the north end of the island, the ground rising steadily. They came around an ascending curve and all at once the lush tropical greenery was gone on the left side, revealing a grand sweep of lawn that flowed up the side of the hill to a building of white and gray.

As they drew closer, Carras saw that it was actually two buildings: one was single-level, a U-shaped structure that seemed almost completely walled in glass, great vertical windows that must be fourteen feet high; the other was a two-story block, with a third, smaller level on top, also walled in glass. It was placed like an accent above the open U of the low-rise.

Between the buildings was a spacious courtyard that looked to be flagged in marble, with a riot of blooming shrubs and creepers in raised beds. As they parked in the gap between the two buildings, Carras saw that much of the U was filled by an oblong of blue water.

Flynnt led him across the courtyard and through an open glass door on the seaward side of the U. There was a lounge, simply but elegantly furnished.

They went through an inner door which led into a succession of rooms—library, billiards, one with a large-screen television—until they came to a corner of the U which looked out over the sea to the east and the full length of the island to the south.

The room had been designed around a heavy mahogany dining table that would seat at least twenty, although only a few chairs were grouped around the far end. A servant in a white jacket was laying out two more place settings of linen and silver to go with the four that were already there, and two other men were bringing in chairs to complement the settings. They finished their work and left silently.

The servants' activity had briefly obscured the presence of the two couples seated at the end of the table. As Flynnt led Carras down past the length of polished dark wood, the doctor saw that one of the men was an East Indian, about thirty, with delicate features and slim hands, dressed in a slightly out-of-fashion suit. The Indian woman who sat beside him was dressed as a nurse. The other man was in his thirties, with the same hair and eyes as Terry Flynnt, though the face was softer. The man was clearly unwell, but Carras could not study him closely, because Flynnt was making introductions.

"This is Philip, my son," Flynnt said, "and his wife, Annabella." Carras instantly recognized the slender, blue-eyed brunette. He had seen her face on the covers of magazines that he never bought, because the contents were exclusively devoted to female fashion. The Indian man was Dr. Ashok Gupta and the nurse was his wife, Ranjit.

When Flynnt identified Carras by name the Indian man said, "I know of your work, doctor."

"You are a medical doctor?" Carras asked, when they were seated.

"I am a cardiologist, formerly with the University of Mumbai, now in attendance on Mr. Flynnt," Gupta said.

Carras took a closer look at Philip. His color was sallow and the veins in his neck were abnormally full. His breathing was shallow, but at regular intervals he sighed deeply, which to Carras meant that his body's precise regulatory mechanisms were trying to extract every molecule of oxygen from the air in his lungs. And he was thin, too thin in his face and extremities, though his waistline was swollen—fluid in the abdomen, Carras thought.

The symptoms were those of either advanced lung disease or end-stage heart failure. The fact that Philip was attended by a cardiologist, not a respiratory specialist, made the diagnosis easy. Carras would have liked to ask a question or two, but this was breakfast, not a consulting room.

Philip said, "Before you came, doctor, we were talking about cars. Dr. Gupta has a misguided affection for the Jaguar."

"I said only that I saw one in Mumbai that belonged to a Bollywood movie star, and it looked very fine," the Indian said.

"You're a formula one racer," Carras said. "I think I've read about you."

"I used to be," Philip said, his voice made soft by his illness. "I was no Andretti, but I could get around the track." He sighed. "An indulgence of a rich man for his son, you might think, but I paid my own way. I even paid for the practice track around the island."

"Your father didn't approve?" Carras asked, looking to Flynnt senior. But the older man showed no response.

"He did not," Philip said. "He believed I should be involved in the family business. I told him I'd be happy to jump right in, but I wanted to do things my way." He shook his head. "Let's not talk about that. How about you, doctor—are you an automobile enthusiast?"

"I have a 1986 De Tomaso Pantera. The GTS with a tweaked engine and suspension."

"Now, that's a car," Philip said.

"It was the only thing in my life that I ever just had to have," Carras said. "I saw one in a Lincoln-Mercury dealer's window in New Haven when I was still an intern at Yale. Fly yellow. I couldn't believe the lines of the thing. It was beautiful. I went home and said to my wife, "When I start making decent money, that's the first thing I'm going to buy.' And it was."

Carras said he'd wound it out on a couple of race tracks that opened on their off days for amateurs. "And my teenage son and I are going to take her down the Pacific Coast Highway this summer, from the Napa Valley to San Diego."

"Tell me about the Pantera," Philip said. "I'm starved for car talk. I've got a 1972 Ferrari Daytona parked in the hangar down at the airstrip."

"I think I'd rather talk about your Ferrari," Carras said. The Daytona convertible was the most beautiful car ever made and the vee-twelve beneath the long hood was a poem in steel.

"I used to drive it on the track to keep in practice," Philip said. "Now I don't use it—my condition, obviously —but..."

"You can't bear to part with it," Carras said. He knew from looking at the sick man that there was slim chance he would ever drive the classic again.

"Yeah," Philip sighed, and not just out of a need for oxygen.

Carras was always willing to talk high-performance cars, so it wasn't just out of sympathy for the sick man that he said, "Well, you've got me on cylinders and revs, but I've got you on cc's and torque."

The Ferrari boasted an elegant vee-twelve Italian engine; the Pantera was a combination of Italian style and American brute force. A professional driver behind the wheel of the Ferrari would probably wax a gifted amateur like Carras off the track, but the Pantera's sheer muscle would let him give a good account of himself.

Carras found himself liking the younger man and felt a wave of tenderness for his wife. It was more than the familiar reaction that rose in him when confronted by the kind of illness he had dedicated his life to alleviating. He felt he would like to know these people just as people, to linger over lunch with them, to take the cars for a spin around the track.

He wanted to ask about Philip's condition, but just then the servants brought in breakfast: a selection of breads and fruits, perfectly fresh, with a bowl of almond flavored home-made yogurt that was simply the best Carras had ever tasted, rich, hot coffee in a carafe and fruit juices. Terry Flynnt ate sparingly, and drank only a concoction that was brought to him alone, its surface piled with blender-generated bubbles. The bike race had left Carras ravenous and he ate well, taking seconds of the yogurt.

He was waiting for the older man to bring the conversation around to what must obviously be the connection between the sick son and the surgeon's presence in this house. But Terry Flynnt said nothing, just sat there chewing methodically as if he were the only one in the room. The car talk continued through the meal.

The Guptas ate quietly, adding little to the conversation, and keeping a close eye on their patient.

"My father had me working on engines when I was six years old," Carras said. "He was a mechanic in the Greek air force, came to America after World War Two and ended up owning a gas station in Philadelphia. If you'd asked me at twelve what I was going to do with my life, I'd have said I was going to keep on doing what I was already doing—fixing cars."

"But you didn't."

"No. My dad said I should go to school, be an engineer. I was accepted to MIT before I was halfway through high school. But then one of my teachers steered a recruiter from Yale my way, they were offering scholarships, and that's where I ended up. I've never left."

Dr. Gupta said, "Dr. Carras is one of the finest cardiothoracic surgeons in the world."

"Really," said Philip, looking at his father, whose attention was fixed on his meal. "Isn't that a coincidence?"

"I have read your book on aneurysectomy," the Indian said to Carras. "Very fine. Also, I closely followed the case of Dr. Goldenberg. It was terribly unfair how you were treated by the press."

"Thank you, doctor," Carras said. "Are you a surgeon?"

Gupta waggled the fingers of one delicate hand. "I am more on the clinician side of things."

"I couldn't help noticing your condition," Carras said to Philip. He looked at the Indian. "Cardiomyopathy?"

Dr. Gupta confirmed the diagnosis.

"Goddamn virus, was all," Philip said. "You think you've got a little cold, next thing you know it's eating your heart out."

It was a layman's description of a rare heart disease that could happen to anyone. A common cold virus had infected Philip's system in the normal way. But instead of being confined to and by the mucous membranes of his respiratory system, this virus had got into his blood stream. Then it had found a tiny but useful crevice somewhere in his heart, staying long enough to enter one of the cardiac muscle cells.

It had chemically perverted the DNA in the nucleus of the cell, turning it into a biological factory to produce more of its own kind. Eventually, the cell was so full of replicated viruses, and so weakened by its unnatural efforts, that its membrane had burst, spewing a flood of viruses onto its sister cells, many of which were penetrated by the pathogens. The process then repeated itself exponentially.

Much of the muscle that made up Philip's heart was now destroyed. There was no cure. The virus was now long gone, but it had so weakened the organ that it could no longer function well enough to sustain the rest of the body's systems. At some point, and it would be soon, Philip would die.

There was no cure, but there was a treatment. "Is there an impediment to your seeking a heart transplant?" Carras asked, thinking as he did that here might be an explanation for the father's interest in him.

Philip shook his head, and Gupta said, "We have not been able to find a donor match. Too many antibodies."

Carras understood that Philip was one of those unfortunate patients whose immune systems were too thoroughly on guard against foreign tissues, even with immunosuppressive drugs. Outside of his own gene pool, it would be rare to find a heart that would match.

The ill young man showed a wan smile. "I have accepted it," he said. "My father calls it giving up. It drives him up the wall."

Annabella looked at her father-in-law and said, "He wouldn't even know where to look in the dictionary to find the definition of giving up."

Flynnt inclined his head slightly and raised his glass of elixir in an ironic salute. It was the first evidence since he had introduced them that he recognized their existence. Beneath Annabella's beauty Carras saw a woman in despair. "I am sorry," he said.

The old man drained his glass, set it down and placed his hands palms down on the table top. *Here it comes*, Carras thought.

But whatever Flynnt was about to say was pre-empted by the chime of a cell phone. For the first time, Carras saw a look of surprise animate the elder Flynnt's face, as he reached into his pocket for the ringing phone. Clearly, the call was unexpected.

"Who is this?" he said, in a tone that promised an unhappy outcome for whoever had called him on this number. But as Carras watched, the billionaire's poker face swiftly reasserted itself. Flynnt listened for a moment then rose and said, "I'll take this in the next room."

Philip and Annabella gave each other looks that said, *Your guess is as good as mine.* The woman turned to Carras and said, "So why has he brought you here, doctor? Do you know that you're the first unfamiliar face in this house since Philip got sick?"

"I've no idea," Carras said, "but he went to an awful lot of trouble." He briefly sketched the business of the grant and Hilary and the research building. "I think that he thinks he's making me an offer I can't refuse, but he hasn't said what he wants."

"So that's what all the busy-busy construction was about," Philip said. "He wouldn't tell us what was going on, and the servants were ordered to stay away."

Annabella said, "I went down, but the security people stopped me on the road and made me turn around."

"Security?" Carras said.

"It's unobtrusive," Annabella said, "but don't try to land a boat or a plane on this island without clearance."

"The business with Hilary Cartiere bothers me," Philip said. "He's turned pretty strange the past few months. But hiring a movie star to draw you into his web is a whole new order of weirdness." He coughed and Carras could see that the effort required merely to conduct a conversation was taking a toll. "I can tell you it's got nothing to do with my illness," he continued when the spasms stopped. "The chances of my finding a compatible heart are one in a million. I'm not expecting any miracles."

"Something good will happen," Annabella said. "I'm not giving up hope."

Gupta spoke. "I think it is time for my patient to rest, doctor." Both he and his wife got up, she going to a side door that turned out to be a closet. She returned with a wheelchair into which Philip was swiftly transferred. "I hope to see you again, doctor," the cardiologist said, as the nurse wheeled the sick man away.

"I don't think the old man's right in the head any more," Annabella said, when she and Carras were alone. "It's Philip's illness. Seeing his only son being slowly struck down before his eyes has made him conscious of his own death. I think he's determined to go on living, no matter what."

"Most people want to go on living, no matter what," Carras said. "It's why many terminal cancer patients live with the misery and sickness of chemotherapy, just to get a few more weeks or months of life."

"With Terry Flynnt, I don't think it's life itself that appeals to him," Annabella said. "I mean, he's living now like some kind of ascetic monk, popping vitamins and pushing himself to the limit. What he wants, all he wants, is to hold on to what he's got. He can't bear the thought of his... his stuff falling into somebody else's hands."

"Is that what he says?"

"It's what I believe."

Her assessment fitted with how Carras had summed up the billionaire's motivations. Flynnt played to win, and he played for keeps. "There's nothing unnatural about that, either," he said. "People who build vast fortunes tend to want to hold onto them."

"Well, I just want you to know who you're dealing with. He's not a man who takes no for an answer."

"How does he take 'impossible?'" Carras said.

"When it's applied to him getting something that he wants, that's another word he doesn't know the meaning of. You should have seen how he reacted when Philip said he wanted to sell his shares in the business."

She told him how, way back when the original Flynnt operation was a private company with one little plastics factory in Ohio, Flynnt had split the shares with his wife, Carol—for tax reasons, Annabella thought. After the company started to grow, the division of ownership remained and when Flynnt went public in the eighties, Philip's mother owned a sizable stake. But she always let the old man have her proxy, so it was as if the shares were his.

The situation didn't change when Carol died. Her will left all of her holdings to their son, and since Philip's only interest in those days was building and racing formula one cars, he left the proxy arrangements as they were. Terry Flynnt always expected his son to grow out of his love affair with the track and step into the family business. But then Philip married Annabella, a woman with a well developed social conscience and a degree from the London School of Economics.

"Philip did grow up, but not the way his father expected. He came to see that there was more to life than getting and spending," she said. "He wanted to do something to help people who can't help themselves. We were talking about selling his shares and creating a trust that would do some good in poor countries, maybe drill wells for clean water in places where half the children die of diarrhea. Or make micro-loans of a few hundred bucks each to women in third world villages so they can start small businesses—making tortillas or weaving cloth—and become independent."

"How did Philip's father react?" Carras said.

"He went kind of nuts. He said if Philip put such a large block of shares on the market, it would drive down the share price. That would make the outside directors on the board very unhappy and weaken the company to the point where they'd be vulnerable to a takeover."

"That sounds like a reasonable worry."

"Maybe," Annabella said. "And if Terry had been more reasonable in his

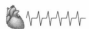

response we could have worked something out. Instead, it was all 'no son of mine,' and 'I will never forgive you.' It was a pretty memorable fight. He called Philip a 'half-assed bleeding-heart crackpot,' and Philip said Terry had the 'ethical sensibilities of a bacterium.' They haven't spoken since."

"Not even after Philip became ill?" Carras said.

She shook her head. "Nope. Terry Flynnt's not a man to talk about his feelings, even if he still has any. Besides, by then we'd gone ahead with our plans, at least the preliminary stages. Then Philip got sick and didn't have the energy to do what we wanted to do. I wasn't going to leave my ailing husband helpless while I went off to save the world. So we let Terry keep the proxy."

"Excuse me for being blunt," Carras said, "but what happens when Philip dies?"

"If Philip goes," she corrected him, "I will inherit his shares. I will withdraw the proxy from the old man and I will create the foundation in my husband's memory."

The determination in her voice caused a chill to pass through Carras. The fairy tale wondrousness of meeting and bedding Hilary Cartiere had fully receded, revealing a background of intrafamily conflict at the heart of which was an immensely powerful man thought by his closest relatives to be "not right in the head." *I do not want to be involved in this*, he thought.

"One thing nobody will tell me is how long Philip has," Annabella said.

"I don't think it would be proper for me to say. He's not my patient. I haven't examined him."

"But you've seen many like him."

"How bad is his shortness of breath?" Carras asked.

"It used to be bad when we took a walk or made love," she said. "Lately, though, he wakes up gasping for breath in the night. We tried to make love a couple of weeks ago. He started to turn blue. He has a device implanted in his chest..."

"A defibrillator?" Carras said.

"Yes," she said. "It kicked in and restored his heart beat."

Carras sighed. "From what you're telling me and from what I've seen, there will have been a back-up of fluid in his lungs, causing the shortness of breath. Sounds like it's been getting worse. I noticed a swollen abdomen— that's more fluid retention. I wish I could offer you hope, but I would say it's time to prepare for..." He spread his hands.

The beautiful face was stark with grief. "If only he could have a transplant."

It was ironic, Carras knew. The same hypervigilant immune system that had defended Philip Flynnt from infections and disease pathogens all his life now produced the antibodies that prevented the only procedure that could save him.

"They've made great advances in artificial hearts," he said. "Any day now, someone could announce a solution to the clotting problem, and that would make it possible for him to wait as long as needed for a compatible donor."

"But it will have to be soon, won't it?" she said. "Really soon."

Carras didn't want to say it. Even when it wasn't his own patient, he hated to admit that death was about to claim a victory.

"Tell me," she said. "I have a right to know."

"It might be only a matter of days."

She nodded. He could see it was what she had expected to hear, dreaded it but knew it was coming. She rose from the table. "I should go to him," she said and went to the door they had wheeled Philip through, turning at the last moment to say, "Excuse me."

"Of course," Carras said.

Terry Flynnt came back into the room. There was no way for Carras to tell from his expression whether the unexpected phone call had been a minor irritation or the end of the world. The surgeon said, "Mr. Flynnt, I thank you for your hospitality, but I would like to leave now."

The old man's impassive face didn't change. "Of course, doctor," he said. "I will tell them to get the plane ready." He punched a button on his cell phone and issued orders. When that was done, he said to Carras, "It will take a few minutes. In the meantime, if you will indulge me, there's one more thing I'd like to show you."

Flynnt and Carras went back down the hill in the Range Rover, then took a road that angled inland, skirting the base of the slope then leading them down to the western coast of the island. They came out of the trees to see a jetty of wooden planks over piled rocks that ran far out into the blue water. At the end of the dock was the largest yacht Carras had ever seen.

Carras was no sailor but he had been on a few yachts. He could see that this boat was something special, easily two hundred feet in length, the size of a small cruise ship. The hull was dark blue, the superstructure glaring white in the tropical sun. The three decks showed a swept-back profile that created the illusion that the yacht was surging forward even while she stood still at the dock. An array of radar and communications masts aft of the bridge looked state of the art. Carras was sure the interior fittings and furnishings would also be the finest money could buy.

That expectation was confirmed when the Range Rover stopped at the seaward end of the jetty and Flynnt led him aboard. They passed through corridors paneled in teak lit by glass fixtures Carras thought must be antique Lalique, with everywhere the gleam of polished brass and rich dark wood. At the end of one hallway, the old man unlocked a door and they descended a companionway.

At the bottom of the stairs was a door and beyond it the luxurious appointments stopped. Here it was tile and paint under fluorescent lights, and a pair of metal doors which Flynnt unlocked with a key that hung from a chain around his neck. Beyond was a surgical scrub room with sterile garments folded in paper wraps. At the other end of the room were two more doors with circular windows.

"Look through there," Flynnt said, and flicked a switch that lit up the space behind the doors.

Carras looked through one of the windows and saw a fully equipped operating theater, complete with heart-and-lung machine and all the paraphernalia needed for cardiac surgery. There were two tables.

Against the far wall was a glass-faced cupboard containing two shiny metal objects that Carras at first couldn't make out, though the shape tickled his memory. A moment later, the answer came. "Those are atomic hearts," he said.

"Right," said Flynnt. "The last two in existence. And before you ask, yes, they do contain plutonium and they are in working order."

Carras knew that Epsilon Pharmaceuticals had developed a plutonium-powered mechanical heart back in the sixties, solving one of the perennial problems of a self-contained artificial organ: the need for an external power supply. A heart, natural or man-made, had to be able to pump five quarts of blood a minute, all day and every day. No battery strong enough for the purpose was small enough to fit inside the human body.

The atomic option had worked splendidly in animal tests. But the US Atomic Energy Commission had ruled out the placement of plutonium in private hands—or more accurately, in private torsos—for fear that terrorists would capture and kill atomic heart recipients and thus assemble enough of the deadly radioactive material to build a nuclear bomb or poison a city's water supply.

"I thought they had all been dismantled," Carras said.

"Epsilon kept two and kept quiet about it," Flynnt said. "But not quiet enough. I bought the company and had them moved down here."

"You can't seriously expect me to put one of those in your son," he said.

Flynnt laughed. It was a short bark and Carras didn't think there was much humor behind it. He heard it as the kind that of laugh that didn't say *That's funny*, so much as it said, *I win*.

"No. A few months ago that would have been the plan. But artificial hearts create clots and clots cause strokes, and that's a problem nobody has solved."

"Then what do you want?"

"I want you to perform a heart transplant on Philip. Here on this yacht."

"You have a compatible donor?"

"I will have."

"Then all you have to do is fly Philip to where the donor is and have the procedure performed. You don't need to pay a billion dollars. You don't need your own operating room."

"Yes, I do," Flynnt said. "Because I want the operation performed here. And I want you to do it."

"Why me?"

"You are the best," Flynnt said. "The Goldenberg case proved that to my satisfaction. I will always have the best."

"It makes no sense," Carras said. "There is no need to go to all this trouble..."—then it struck him—"unless the operation is illegal."

"It will be technically illegal," Flynnt said. "But it will be performed on this ship while we are in international waters."

"What does that mean?"

"It means," said Flynnt, "that you will be governed by the laws of the country in which the ship is registered. In this case, that happens to be Liberia, and these days Liberia is about as close to a country without laws as you can get."

"I won't perform an illegal procedure," Carras said.

Flynnt ignored his refusal.

For Carras, the discussion was over. He wanted to get on the jet and go away from this man and his island and his assumption that everything would go the way he said it would.

Flynnt said, "I have assembled a full team of qualified people to assist you. They'll be here in a couple of days. There will be a transplant. And there will be a compatible donor."

The quiet certainty in Flynnt's voice brought the chill back to Carras's spine. Worldwide, there were millions of potentially compatible donors even for antibody resistant cases like Philip's. It was just rare for one of them to be pronounced brain dead in a hospital within four hours flight time from where the patient happened to be.

"Murder is a crime, Mr. Flynnt," he said, "even in Liberia. If you're thinking I will kill some poor soul who happens to have the right blood and tissue types, you're as crazy as your daughter-in-law thinks you are."

Again came the humorless bark of laughter. "The donor is willing," Flynnt said.

The implications of what the man was saying horrified Athan Carras. Someone was going to give his life to save Philip's. Some dirt-poor Filipino fisherman or Central American farmer with ten sick kids he couldn't support had hit the Terry Flynnt tissue-type lottery. *Here you go, Third World Dad,* he thought, *here's enough money for your kids to go to school and live like human beings. Just lie down and let one of the world's best cardiothoracic surgeons cut out your heart.*

"Who?" he said.

"You don't need to know that," Flynnt said.

"Does Philip know what you're planning to do? Or Annabella?"

"They do not."

"They deserve to know."

Flynnt shook his head. "They would not approve."

"I want to talk to them," Carras said.

"No."

"Then I want to leave," he told the billionaire. "Right now."

• • •

Terry Flynnt turned to watch the jet carrying the surgeon and the movie star roll down the runway. Isaac stood beside the Range Rover until the plane lifted off, then he opened the door and the billionaire climbed in.

Flynnt said, "I had a call on my private number this morning. Find out how the number was compromised and make sure it doesn't happen again."

"Yes, sir," Isaac said. "You want to tell me who it was?"

"Who do you think?"

Isaac put the vehicle into gear and they drove back to the yacht. Flynnt turned to watched the plane dwindle into a bright speck of reflected sunlight. The doctor had wanted to turn down the offer on the spot, but Flynnt had told the man that he would not accept an answer now. In two days the rest of the transplant team would be on the island. Then Flynnt would send Maigrot and Isaac for Carras.

But the call at breakfast had been an unwelcome reminder that other forces might begin to change the timetable Flynnt had set.

When Flynnt had answered the phone with Who is this?, the voice that had come through the cell phone's ear piece had had a western twang behind the vowels. It was a voice that had probably started out rough, and years of whiskey and cigars had made it even rougher. "This is Victor Whitehall," it said. "We should talk."

Flynnt had gotten up from the breakfast table and gone to another room before he said, "About what?"

"I think you know."

Flynnt said nothing. It was the other man's ball to play and he didn't see why he should help set it up for him.

After a moment, Whitehall said, "I hear you've been on your yacht in Miami. I'm coming down there. Why don't we get together?

"I don't see the need," Flynnt said.

"Maybe I can help you see it," Whitehall said. "I'll be in touch."

The Range Rover rumbled over the wooden jetty. "What did you think of the doctor?" Flynnt asked Isaac.

"Man cuts people's hearts out, he's got to have some balls."

"You think it's no?"

"I think it's no," Isaac said.

"Did we play him wrong?"

"I think maybe so."

"The bike race?"

"He didn't like losing."

Flynnt made a noise with his tongue and teeth. "What then?"

Isaac shrugged. "Get somebody else."

"No, he's the one. But we're running out of time."

Isaac said, "Well, we showed him some heaven. I was thinking maybe we need to give him some hell."

Flynnt said, "That's what I was thinking. After I talked to Whitehall, I called our friend the banana grower."

Isaac nodded, remembering. "It worked when we caught that guy from the industrial espionage firm. A few days on the plantation, he told us everything."

"I gave the doctor two days to think it over. Is that enough time to set it up?"

"No problem."

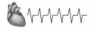

Chapter 8

Hilary Cartiere was twenty-two-year-old Hilda McCarty when she arrived in Los Angeles in the early seventies. She had an average talent but better than average looks, in an industry where the average is set very high.

She signed with a low-rent talent agency and went to open-call auditions. Soon she was doing what most "starlets" had to do to get small roles—blow-jobs for bit-parts, her roommates called it. But she was determinedly working her way up. At first she was just a face in a crowd scene; then she started being singled out for reaction shots, gasping or screaming to punctuate a piece of action. Soon, she was given a line or two of dialogue and those few seconds of celluloid almost never ended up on an editor's floor.

Even indifferently lit, her face drew the eye. She had a luminous quality on screen, a natural presence that appeared the moment the camera caught her, adding something indefinably magical to her already attractive features.

A big-name director saw it first in the daily rushes of a romantic comedy. She played a waitress in a French cafe—her only line was, "Coffee, *m'sieur, madame?*"—while the romantic leads ignored her and stared into each other's eyes. When the director saw Hilary on film, he had the writers add a little bit of business between her and the male star and reshot the scene.

The movie previewed at a theater in Pasadena. Sid Hoffman, a partner in one of the top agencies, took one look at Hilary Cartiere's thirty-second showcase and went to the phone in the lobby. By ten a.m. the next morning he had her signature on a contract.

Two years later, she was one of the most bankable female leads in the industry. The fees got bigger and the parts got better as the seventies became the eighties. Hilary threw herself into the whirlwind of a star's life, living every moment to the full, and spending almost every penny she earned. But in the nineties, the parts got smaller, the phone didn't ring so often. She was short-listed for some serious dramatic parts but always seemed to lose out to Meryl Streep or Faye Dunaway or Sigourney Weaver.

She sat beside her pool one afternoon, contemplating reality: she hadn't worked in five years, her money was almost gone and the only part she was asked to read for was playing a wacky washed-up movie star, the neighbor of some stand-up comic in a lame sit-com pilot.

Sid was urging her to take it. She got the clear impression that when he retired, and it wouldn't be long before that happened, none of his younger partners would be leaping to pick up her business.

"Oh, god," she said to the empty patio, "one good part and I could make it work again. One good picture."

It was then that the phone rang and Leonard Maigrot asked if she would be available to meet with his employer. It had been a long time since anyone had sent a jet for her. She was there the same day.

In the villa, she'd told Athan Carras that she wouldn't have agreed to do just anything with just anyone for guaranteed financing of a comeback picture. She was sure that was the truth, although she couldn't think of an example where she would have actually drawn the line.

"I want you to be nice to a man who needs someone to be nice to him," Flynnt had said. "And you're the perfect someone."

It hadn't been hard to be nice to Athan Carras. He'd been sweet, a genuine fan and she didn't meet so many of those any more. As a lover she would place him somewhere in the middle of the pack, but—whatever this had all been about—if it came down to a contest of wills between the doctor and the billionaire, she'd put her money on Terry Flynnt.

She was having breakfast on the Boeing when Carras came aboard. The blonde steward offered Carras a champagne and orange juice cocktail, but he waved her away.

"Is something wrong?" Hilary said.

"I think so, very wrong," Carras said. He told her that Flynnt wanted him to perform an illegal operation. He seemed genuinely upset.

"What did you say?" she asked.

"I told him I'm not for sale."

"Wow," she said. "Are you sure you don't want a cocktail? You look like you could use a drink."

"No," he said. "No booze."

"Do you want to talk about it?"

He looked at her with real worry on his face. "I better not. It could be trouble for you, if you know about this."

She felt a twinge of concern for the man. He seemed genuinely upset. But she couldn't let anything screw up her comeback deal. "If that's the way you feel," she said.

They didn't talk all the way back to Miami. He stared out the window and brooded. When they touched down at the airport and taxied to a stop, he stood up and was waiting at the door when the attendant opened it and the ground crew pushed the stairway into place. Hilary thought he seemed impatient to get somewhere.

Carras left the plane immediately, but a moment later he came back through the door. "Aren't you coming?" he said.

Hilary was still seated on the couch. "No, sweetie," she said. "I've got a lot of work waiting for me in LA."

"But I thought..."

She shook her head, the same way she'd shaken it in *Fire River.* "Call me," she said.

"Sir," the stewardess said, "We have to leave or we'll lose our place in the take-off rotation."

"Call me," Hilary said again.

"I will," Carras said, confusion on his face as the young woman gently but firmly set him on his way down the stairs.

The jet's rear door closed and the engines' whine increased in pitch. Hilary watched through the window as Carras got into the car that was waiting for him. The vehicle sped away immediately.

While the Boeing taxied back out to the runway, Hilary asked the attendant to bring her another champagne cocktail. She wondered how long it would take the doctor to realize that she had never given him her number. Then she sighed and put him out of her mind while she concentrated on what she would need to do once she was back in LA, and back in business.

• • •

In the car taking him back to the Loews Hotel, Carras turned on his cell phone and checked his voice mail. Charlie Vance had left three messages and his own cell number.

"What the hell happened to you?" Vance said when Carras got him on the phone.

"I'll tell you when I see you."

"Okay, have lunch in my room. I've got something to show you."

Lunch was steak for Vance, an omelet for Carras, and before it arrived the surgeon gave his friend the highlights of the past twenty-four hours.

"Hilary Cartiere?" Vance said. "You were honest-to-god banging Hilary Cartiere?" He was of the same generation as Carras, had had the same poster.

Carras had never been comfortable with locker-room sex talk. "That's not the important part," he said.

"Says you."

Carras told Vance about the breakfast with Philip and Annabella and the operating room on the yacht. "Ah," said Vance, when he heard about the younger Flynnt's cardiomyopathy, "that fills in a blank."

"What do you mean?"

There was a knock on the door. The food had arrived, and Carras had to wait until the meal was set up and signed for before he could repeat the question.

Vance cut himself a cubic inch of rare porterhouse and chewed with vigor, eyebrows dancing. He swallowed and reached over to the bed and picked up a file folder stuffed with paper. "Check this out," he said and cut another cube of meat.

Carras let his meal go cold as he began to look through the thick sheaf of paper his friend handed him.

"Remember Mike the corporate headhunter?" Vance said. "I had his research department pull whatever they had on Terry Flynnt and e-mail it down to me. Not bad, eh?"

Carras thumbed through the material. There were magazine articles, brokerage house reports, some e-mails marked Confidential and the chairman's remarks sections from a couple of recent annual reports of the Flynnt Group of companies. "I want to read this," he said.

"I already have," Vance said. "Eat your food and I'll tell you what it's all about."

Terry Flynnt had started out with a small factory in Ohio that made plastic coatings for all kinds of consumer goods. "He inherited the place from his father, who died young not long after Terry got his degree in chemical engineering," Vance said. "The old man was a drunk, but it seems young Terry was brilliant."

After his father's death in the late sixties, the company took off. Flynnt put together a little research shop and began experimenting with exotic compounds. "You know the stuff they paint ships and stealth bombers with, so they absorb radar instead of bouncing it back? He was a pioneer there, got some patents that must have paid billions."

"Then he stepped out a little and bought some other companies," Vance said, "but carefully. Always stuck to his knitting, bought operations that fit closely with what he was already doing. Soon you practically couldn't make a tank or a fighter or a camouflage suit without buying some crucial component from the Flynnt Group. The Reagan-Bush years were very, very good to Terry Flynnt."

Then in the late eighties, the Flynnt Group had gone public to raise capital for larger-scale military systems. "Amazingly," Vance said, "they all worked as specified."

Today, Flynnt controlled a tightly connected group of manufacturing companies with a seven-member board of directors. Terry Flynnt was chair and chief executive officer of the corporate group. His son Philip, by virtue of his personal share of the corporation's stock, had a seat. There was a retired major general who was on the board solely for his very useful Pentagon contacts, and there were three directors, all accountants by profession, who answered to the pension and mutual funds that had taken substantial positions in the Flynnt Group when it had gone public.

"But there's a newcomer to the board," Vance continued. "His name is Arthur Pennock, a corporate lawyer, and he was nominated to the board at the last annual general meeting by a new significant shareholder: the Whitehall Holdings Corporation."

Buying on the open market, Whitehall had acquired eight per cent of Flynnt Group shares, a mix of common and preferred, enough to get his nominee on the board. Now, the confidential e-mails said, Whitehall was trying to purchase more of the conglomerate's stock, all he could get his hands on. "He must have heard that Philip was ill," Vance said.

"Or maybe just that he was thinking of setting up his charitable foundation," Carras said.

Either way, Whitehall was acquiring Flynnt Group shares. When he had enough, he would push to get another of his people around the board table, then his directors would exert influence on the fund representatives and the retired general. "It's his standard operating procedure, according to Mike," Vance said.

"So Flynnt, though he holds the largest block of shares and Philip holds the second, could lose control of the company he built up from the little plant his wastrel father left him.

"Flynnt would still be one of the richest men in the world, a billionaire several times over," Vance continued. "In fact, the fight for control would drive up the price of his shares and make him even richer."

"For guys like him, it's not about the money," Carras said. "It's about winning. If Philip dies his shares go to a foundation. Its directors would probably sell to Whitehall, because they'd make a big capital gain and that would increase the value of the trust. And Flynnt would have been beaten by this Whitehall guy."

"You think so?" Vance said. "Maybe he really cares about his son."

"I met the guy, Charlie," Carras said, "saw him with Philip. He didn't speak one word to him."

"Sometimes fathers find it difficult to talk to sons, especially when there's been a breach. With death in the picture, it could make it even harder."

His friend's words rang a faint bell somewhere inside Athan Carras. He thought about how hard it had been to talk to Costas on the phone. But he rejected the comparison. Flynnt was a hard man in a hard world. That was all there was to it.

Vance was still talking. "Mike's broker has heard rumors about Flynnt selling off some of his shares, building up liquidity. That had Mike puzzled. Now it makes sense—well, a kind of sense. He was putting together the fund he offered you."

"Which I'm not going to accept," Carras said. "Because the only thing I can think of is he's also offered money to some poor bastard who's going to give up his heart. And there's no way I'm killing a man—willing volunteer or no—so that Terry Flynnt can beat this Whitehall."

Vance poured them some coffee. "It raises an interesting philosophical question, though. It's one I've discussed with my students many a time—does a man have a right to end his own life for a good cause?"

"How is preserving Flynnt's financial empire a good cause?"

"Not that. But suppose there is some Filipino farmer who's willing to sell his heart to lift his family out of poverty. We say that's wrong. But if he's willing to put in forty years working himself to death just to keep them in rice and rags, we say that's a noble life."

"It's wrong to kill people, even people who are willing to die," Carras said. "It's murder."

"You're against physician-assisted suicide? Even for terminal patients in terrible pain?"

It was an issue that had troubled Carras enough to drive him to research it. "I happen to have seen a court judgment on that question. The Eighth Circuit Court found that the right to life is protected under the right to privacy—depriving someone of life is the ultimate deprivation of privacy. They ruled that physician-assisted suicide is unconstitutional."

"I remember the ruling," Vance said. "I also remember that it wasn't unanimous."

"Do you side with the minority?"

"I'm just arguing the question," said Vance. "It's what philosophers are paid for. How about this one: when we send soldiers into battle we expect them to be willing to die for their country or their buddies."

Carras always liked to argue with the ethicist. It kept him sharp. "That's different," he said. "They're risking their lives, not throwing them away. We don't admire the Japanese kamikaze pilots."

"Our guys at the Alamo went there knowing they were probably going to die. We call them heroes."

"All right," said Carras, "I'll give you a counter example. The tragedy by Euripides, *Alcestis*. The wife dies so that her husband the king may live. But her sacrifice destroys him; he can't bear to live knowing that she gave her life for him. His life has become a death."

"What about the Biblical argument?" Vance said. "Greater love hath no man than this, that he lay down his life for his friends. That's John 13. If it's a blessed thing to die for your friends, how much more blessed is it to die for your loved ones?"

"If Flynnt's plan is what I think it is, we're not talking about dying to save a loved one's life, but about dying to buy them a house in the suburbs," Carras said.

"To be born into poverty is a death sentence," Vance said, "especially in a Calcutta street or a Brazilian slum."

"You can't just limit the discussion to the individual involved," Carras said. "If Flynnt can buy a life and get away with it, more will follow. Letting people commit suicide to sell their organs, for whatever the cause, would open a Pandora's box we might never be able to close."

Vance mulled it a while and said, "I don't know, Ath. Advances in medicine are creating ethical questions that our ancestors never had to ask. It wasn't that long ago that heart transplants were condemned as murder because the donors are technically still alive when their hearts are harvested."

"They're brain dead," Carras said.

"Yeah, but back then brain dead wasn't considered dead enough."

Carras finished his coffee. "It doesn't matter. I'm not going to work for Terry Flynnt. I don't like the arrogance of the man. He can find himself another surgeon."

Vance stuck out his lower lip. "Again, I have to say I don't know, Ath. The way Mike the head hunter tells it, nobody's ever heard of a case of Terry Flynnt not getting whatever he went after. And if he's under pressure from an even bigger son of a bitch like Whitehall..." He sipped coffee and gave Carras an impression of Jack Nicholson facing the inevitable.

Carras said, "He can't pull this kind of crap. Don't we have laws?"

Vance said, "What crap? I'm no lawyer, but I don't think there's any statute against using movie stars to lure doctors to a tropical paradise. And what he said about ships in international waters rings true."

"You think he's expecting me to say yes?" Carras said.

"It's what he's used to hearing."

"But I'm going to say no."

Vance made his eyes and cheeks bulge then said, "Well, that could make things tricky."

"You think he's dangerous." It wasn't a question.

"After what you've told me I think he's nuts," Vance said. "I was already damn sure he was dangerous."

"What do I do?"

"First we drink some more coffee," Vance said. "Then we'll go see a friend of mine who works for the FBI."

• • •

Vance's Cessna 182 was parked at an airfield not far up the coast. Carras squeezed himself into the right-hand seat and buckled up while his friend performed the preflight outside check before climbing in beside him.

"You should learn to fly one of these," Vance said, flicking on the plane's electrical power then pushing in the rod that controlled the fuel mixture. "It goes about twice the speed of your vaunted Pantera."

"Doesn't feel that way," Carras said, "and the roads are a lot smoother than the air you fly through."

Vance turned the ignition switch left then right, then left again. The engine ground and caught. The throttle was halfway out as the pilot spoke to the tower via the hands-free mike and headset and received clearance for take-off. They taxied out to the beginning of the runway then Vance pulled the throttle out to full, holding the plane steady by pressing the tips of the pedals that served as both brake and rudder controls. The propeller spun up to a speed that made it almost invisible and the small aircraft shuddered.

Conversation was impossible. Carras opened the file on Flynnt that Vance had given him and read a few more lines, then he was pushed back into his seat as his friend let go the brakes and the Cessna surged forward.

The little plane didn't need much runway. Within seconds the wheels were bouncing on the pavement and Vance eased the yoke back, lifting them into the air. "You'd like this," he shouted over the rush of air and engine noise. "When I get her up, you should take the yoke."

Carras waved his hand in a gesture that said *no thanks* and kept on reading. One of the Flynnt Group's annual reports contained a listing of products and markets. The interrelated companies sold everything from swamp boots for the Honduran border patrol to plastic bullets for Haitian riot squads. There was scarcely a country in the western hemisphere that Flynnt didn't do business with.

But it wasn't the text that interested Carras: it was the picture on the facing page which showed the corporate group's key officers. There was Terry Flynnt as CEO and Leonard Maigrot identified as Executive Vice President,

Special Projects." And at the end of the back row was the coffee-colored face of Isaac Dumoulin, with the title of "Director of Security."

Carras showed the photo to Charlie Vance. "I met this guy," he shouted. Vance told him to put on a head set so they could talk over the plane's intercom.

"I met this guy," Carras said again, "but I thought he was just the chauffeur."

"Uh uh," said Vance. "There's a write-up on him somewhere in there. He's been with Flynnt since the beginning. Take the yoke."

While Carras gingerly held the twin black plastic handles that controlled the plane's pitch, Vance took the file and hunted through it. "Here," he said, handing Carras a sheet of paper, "it's in the e-mails."

Carras relinquished the yoke and read. It was one of a series of background papers on key decision-makers in the Flynnt Group, the kind of information an executive placement agency routinely prepared on people they might want to approach if a rival corporation hired the head-hunters to raid a competitor's talent.

"He's definitely not just the chauffeur," Carras agreed. Isaac Dumoulin had been eighteen when he volunteered for the US Army in 1968, but he hadn't gone to Vietnam. Instead, after basic training he had been assigned to clerical duties in the Pentagon. The report said that his intelligence and aptitude scores put him in the top percentile, and he had been singled out for special training and advancement—the Army was then beginning to fast-track promising non-white recruits.

He'd spent six years in uniform, along the way leaping the gap between enlisted man and commissioned officer. But in 1974, he'd resigned from a captaincy in a procurement office even though a major's insignia was not far down the track. He'd gone to work for Terry Flynnt and had never left.

"That's interesting," Carras said. "He's on his way to a good career, but he drops it to go work for Terry Flynnt. Why the switch?"

"Check the footnote," Vance said.

Carras looked at the bottom of the report. The footnote said that although there were no records to confirm it, there was a rumor that before going into the army Isaac Dumoulin worked for Flynnt's father at the original factory in Ohio. So had Isaac's mother.

"That shouldn't mean anything," Carras said. "Your average factory hand doesn't act like a loyal family retainer. Flynnt wasn't that big a name in 1974 and Isaac was on track to be a general. He gave up a lot."

"Must like the boss," Vance said. "A lot."

They landed at an airport in Virginia, well outside the security zone that surrounded the District of Columbia and took a cab to the J. Edgar Hoover Building on E Street. The lobby was crowded with high school students waiting to take a tour of the Bureau's anti-crime museum, but when they gave their names to a guard in a glassed-in security booth, they were directed through a metal detector and to a side door that led into a waiting room.

A couple of minutes later, the inner door opened and Vance introduced to Carras to a tall and stooped agent named Fletcher Tully.

"Hear you've had some excitement," Tully said.

"We're more interested in making sure Ath avoids any future thrills and chills," Vance said.

They went upstairs and followed a few corners to a small office where the scattered newspapers on the end table and the spines of books in the bookcase were mostly lettered in Arabic script.

"Fletch helps keep an eye on any would-be jihadists," Vance said.

"So you're not up to date on black-market organs," Carras said.

"I can't even play the piano," the agent said.

"I'm afraid Agent Tully got his sense of humor the same place I got mine," Vance said. "Seriously, Fletch, we're worried that Ath might get dragged into something bad, really bad."

"Sorry," Tully said. "Why don't you tell me the whole thing from the beginning?"

Carras told him. The FBI man listened, made a few notes, asked a few questions. When he got to the part about Hilary Cartiere, Carras had the feeling that Tully had to restrain himself from pressing for the same kind of details Vance had wanted to hear.

After Carras finished his tale, Tully twisted his mouth sideways then said, "I'm not hearing that any crime has been committed. And if there had been, it wouldn't have been committed on US territory." Carras started to say something, but the agent held up a hand. "Now, hold on there, doc. A lot of us FBI agents started out as lawyers, so we tend to think out loud. Flynnt didn't say that he had hired someone to donate his heart?"

"No," Carras said. "That was my assumption."

"Well, if he has, and assuming that the donor is going to kill himself, about the worst you could charge Flynnt with would be assisting a suicide." Tully pulled on his nose while he thought further. "And if that happened on a Liberian registered ship in international waters... I don't even know if Liberia has a law against assisted suicide, but I sure know there wouldn't be a concerted rush to enforce it."

"You're saying he could get away with it," Carras said.

"Like I say, I'm no expert on this kind of thing, but for all we know he wouldn't be the first." The agent picked up his desk phone. "I know somebody you should talk to," he said and punched buttons.

They went up a few floors and down more corridors then through a door into an office much like Tully's but with law books in the bookcases and legal journals on the coffee table. They were introduced to Special Agent Frank Mendoza, a slim man whose hooded eyes and a dark suit gave him the look of a seventeenth-century Jesuit. Carras told his tale for a third time that day.

Mendoza shook his head and confirmed Tully's assessment of the situation. "There wouldn't be a case for us. And we have to be realistic—Liberia's a country without a real government."

"There's another consideration," Charlie Vance said. "Ath has told the man he won't do the operation."

"So he'll find someone who will," Tully said.

Carras shook his head. "My impression is that he's a guy who means to get what he wants. Exactly what he wants."

"You're scared of him," Tully said. It was not a question.

"Anybody in his right mind would be," Carras said.

"But Ath sure as hell is not going to be lured back onto that yacht," Vance added.

Mendoza opened his heavy lidded eyes wider. "You're thinking he might resort to kidnaping?"

"That would get us into the game," Tully said. "If you disappear in the next little while, we'll get a warrant and take a look on that boat, international waters or no."

"If a crime is committed against a US citizen in international waters, we have jurisdiction," Mendoza said.

"You don't understand," Carras said. "If Flynnt is thinking of snatching me, that's not a crime I want you to solve. It's one I want you to prevent."

The agents looked at each other. "Well," said Tully, "the problem is at this point all you've got is a fear of being kidnaped. He didn't threaten to do it, did he?"

"No."

"And when you said you wanted to leave the island, he didn't attempt to confine you unlawfully?"

"No."

Tully shrugged. "Again, it's not my specialty, but you don't appear to have any reasonable apprehension of being snatched." He looked at Mendoza, who shook his narrow head. "So I don't think the Connecticut field office would do—could do—anything at this point. The man has his rights, and you want to be blunt, he's not without power."

"So I'm supposed to just sit and wait for him to come and get me?"

The agents looked at each other again and Carras felt a sinking feeling. Then Mendoza said, "You could buy a panic button, one of those security services that brings a rapid response. Battered women use them."

"What good would that do?"

"Well, if you contracted with the security service to report your disappearance to the Bureau's field office, we'd get that warrant and check the boat."

Carras's temper was beginning to fray. "By the time you get to Flynnt's yacht I could be a mile underneath it."

"I'm sorry," Tully said.

Flying north to New Haven, Carras said, "What am I going to do?"

"You can at least do what Mendoza recommended," Vance said. "Get a panic button service, then call his guy Maigrot. Maybe if you let Flynnt know you were prepared and had talked to the FBI, it might back him off."

Carras nodded without much conviction. "Maybe. Or it just might make him more determined. I'm not sure all his boxcars are connected to the locomotive."

• • •

Leonard Maigrot put down the phone and took the time to make sure his voice had just the right tone—mild puzzlement, no anxiety—before saying, "That was Dr. Carras. He wanted me to know that he's installed a panic button and filed a report with the FBI."

He was in his corner office at the Flynnt Group corporate headquarters, with the view of the scar where the World Trade Center towers used to be. From the leather couch beneath the Monet watercolor Isaac Dumoulin smiled and said, "Good of the man to let us know."

"He thinks we're planning to kidnap him," Maigrot said, and wished the undertone of laughter he'd tried to put beneath the words sounded more convincing.

"Yeah," Isaac said. "How about that?"

Leonard Maigrot had done many questionable things in the service of the Flynnt Group. He had perjured himself in testimony before regulatory bodies. He had suborned public officials, elected and appointed. He had taken part in industrial espionage operations that could probably have been construed as theft of intellectual property. He had made genteel phone calls whose import, as in the case of Carras's Fallon Foundation grant, was nothing less than extortion.

But the worst any of that could have got him was a few months in a country club jail for white-collar offenders. That was a long way from landing in a federal penitentiary, sharing a cell and a toilet with some tattooed, shaven-headed sociopath who'd been longing for a new hobby. He waited for Terry Flynnt's chief of security to say something that would ease his mind. When the seconds ticked away and nothing came, Maigrot said, "Wait a minute."

But Isaac only looked at him until Maigrot looked away.

• • •

There was no listing for Hilary Cartiere in the LA phone book. Carras tried a listing in Van Nuys for a Hilda McCarty but the woman who answered

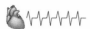

had a thick Irish accent. He remembered that Hilary had mentioned a Sid Hoffman as her agent. A quick search over the Internet produced a slew of references to the name in association with an LA talent agency with an address on Wilshire Boulevard.

The woman who answered also had a pronounced accent, though this one was very, very British. She sounded as if she would be completely at ease taking tea with the queen. No, Mr. Hoffman was not available but she would give him a message if the caller would care to inform her as to the nature of the inquiry. No, she could not provide a telephone number for Ms. Cartiere. Was this is relation to a motion picture project? "No? Then thank you, goodbye."

Carras wondered if his friend Charlie might have one of those handshake connections to someone who knew someone who would know someone who knew Hilary Cartiere. Now that he thought of it, Carras could probably break his own trail to her; he had operated on enough celebrities whose roots were sunk into the entertainment industry.

But even as his hand reached for the address book he kept in a side drawer of the small desk he used when working at home, he stopped. The sun-drenched idyll with the most beautiful woman in the world, the things they'd done and said, were now framed in his mind by the darker reality that Terry Flynnt had set around their moments together. He wondered now how much of it had been a combination of her acting skills and his desire to believe in the magic of it all.

The thought touched a note of sadness inside him and he put it out of his mind. It was better to leave it alone. That way he could let it be what he had wanted it to be, and if it hadn't really been that way, if it had all been an act, he wouldn't have to look at it square on.

He didn't need the address book to dial the number he called instead. The voice that answered was Costas's. When he heard the boy say hello, Carras felt a pang of longing for all the years he had missed, but he kept his tone light and breezy. "How are you doing?"

"Okay." Costas's sounded wary.

"How's school?"

Now the voice warmed a little. "I got an A-plus on my term project, and this prof doesn't hand out many of them."

"Good man!"

"He said I should be talking to a patent attorney."

"No kidding? That is great. I'm proud of you."

"Yeah, well, we'll see."

There was a silence, then Carras said, "So, have you just about wrapped up the term?"

"Yeah, just about."

"Good, cause I'm not doing anything and I was thinking I should get the Pantera shipped out there now and we could take that road trip."

Another silence, this time broken by Costas. "Yeah, all right."

"Great! I'll do it tomorrow."

"Okay."

"Give my love to your mom, and I'll be there in a few days."

"Yeah, okay."

"I'm looking forward to this."

"Me too."

He'd sounded like he meant it, Carras thought when he'd hung up. He called a shipping firm he'd dealt with before and arranged to take the Pantera around to their depot the next day. There wasn't much else to do. He'd put his DHCA student assistants on a literature search pending the approval of his grant application. If Fallon wasn't going to come through, there were other places to look for funds but it would be a while before he could get started.

He thought about driving the Pantera down the Pacific Coast Highway. That would be good; he'd make a clean new start with Costas. It would be slow and difficult to begin with, but it would happen.

Then he thought about when they got to Los Angeles, how they could get a map of the stars' homes and maybe look up Hilary Cartiere. What would Costas think about meeting a real live movie star?

He called Karen. "I'm going to ship the car out west and go see my son," he said. "I don't know when I'll be back."

"Fine. Anything particular you want me to do? Check on your research students?"

"No, they'll be all right. Why don't you take a few days off yourself?"

She had a sister she wanted to visit up in Canada. Carras told her to go ahead and not to record it as part of her regular vacation time.

"You're the boss," she said.

He'd already had the panic button installed, had got onto a security service as soon as he and Vance got back to New Haven. There was a button in the living room and another beside his bed. He'd had a stronger lock installed on the door to the hall and had the slip-and-slide locks on the windows replaced with models that the locksmith recommended.

Now he activated the system and tapped the button in the living room three times to trigger the test sequence that the security firm had recommended he run every now and then. Almost immediately the phone rang and a computerized voice said he had ten seconds to speak a four-digit code. Carras spoke the numbers clearly and the computer thanked him and hung up.

He went out for dinner, carrying the third button: a mobile unit with a built-in digital phone connection. He did not go down to the apartment block's phone room and so he did not see the small electronic device attached to his phone line. Nor did he know that the four digits he had spoken to the security firm's computer were now on a tape recorder in the pocket of Isaac Dumoulin, along with Carras's travel plans.

• • •

The Pantera was safely cocooned in a shipping container that Carras watched being hoisted onto the flatbed of a semi-trailer. Carras then stayed to see that the broad canvas belts that secured the one to the other were tight. He took a cab back to his apartment block to pack a suitcase. He'd decided to travel out west by train, relaxing in a compartment, reading a few books and readying himself to get to know his son again.

He worked the new lock on his door and let himself into the apartment, bolting it securely behind him. Then he walked down the short hallway that separated the living room from the kitchen, heading for the bedroom where his suitcase sat in a closet. As he passed the door to the living room, a nasal voice said, "In here, doctor."

Leonard Maigrot was sitting in his overstuffed armchair, the panic button on the table beside him.

"What the hell are you doing in my apartment?" Carras said.

The downturned mouth twitched. The man was nervous, Carras saw. "We need to talk."

Carras wasn't taking any more of this. He wasn't afraid of this round shouldered, pot-bellied man. "No, we don't. You just need to get the hell out of here."

"No need for emotion," Maigrot said. "My employer sent me..."

"Your employer is either nuts or a criminal or both," Carras said. "And he can't buy me, not even for a billion dollar research endowment."

Carras saw that the number came as a surprise to Leonard Maigrot. "You didn't know about that, did you?" he said.

Maigrot shrugged. "I know what I need to know."

Carras was not fooled. "Well, now you know that my answer is a definite no," Carras said. "I'll spell it for you. F-U-C..."

Carras heard a tiny noise. He turned and saw Isaac in the doorway to the hall, almost filling it. He'd been waiting in the kitchen.

"Look," Carras said to the security chief. "I've got the impression you're a decent man. Do you know what your boss wants me to do?"

There was a flicker of something in the man's eyes. "Yes," Isaac said, "I do."

"Can you be part of that and live with yourself?"

Carras saw by Isaac's face that the question was being taken seriously. "He's doing what he has to. That's all any of us can ever do."

"It's wrong."

Again he saw the tiniest wince, but the words that followed countermanded whatever Isaac was feeling. "It's necessary."

"No," Carras said. He spun and leapt toward the panic button. He expected Maigrot to try to stop him, but the executive reacted with pure fright and dove out the way.

Carras slapped the alarm button. "In a few minutes, men with guns are going to be here," he said.

"I don't think so," said Isaac.

The phone rang. Carras smiled. Isaac nodded to Maigrot. The thin faced man's hand shook as he picked it up and listened. When Maigrot spoke the first digit of the all-clear code Carras threw himself at him, again seeing the look of fear on the man's face.

But somehow Carras's feet were swept out from under him, a heavy weight crashed onto his back and something that felt like a cloth-covered bar of iron went around his neck. The heel of a hard hand pushed against the back of his head, allowing no relief of the pressure the arm was placing on the carotid arteries on either side of his throat. He knew exactly what was being done to him—a classic choke hold that would render him unconscious in seconds. He heard Maigrot's shaky voice finishing the sequence of numbers then the darkness came up and took him.

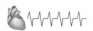

Chapter 9

V ictor Whitehall seldom thought back to his boyhood on a hard-scrabble Oklahoma farm that was blowing away in the dust bowl thirties, but when he did he remembered the pigs. Hard little eyes sunk in folds of thick skin, watching him through the wire fence when he was small and his old man telling him, "Don't you never go in with them hogs, and if you ever go in with 'em, don't you never fall down, cause they'll eatcha fore you kin get up, sure as apples."

He saw them get a little bantam hen that fluttered in to peck at some bugs, three of them zeroing in so fast the chicken was in bloody pieces and going down their throats, feet and all, before it let off more than one surprised squawk, the other pigs rushing over too late to crowd in. The hogs that got nothing squealed a high-pitched excited sound, but from the ones whose mouths were full and rimmed with pink foam came only the crack of breaking bones and that satisfied throat sound that pigs make when they're getting what they want.

But it wasn't any sight or sound that Victor Whitehall remembered first and most; it was the smell of pig shit. The way it got far up into his nose in summer so he thought it was filling all the blank spaces inside him. The way it filled every corner of the house, even when the doors and windows were shut and the wind was blowing the other way. In winter it stank even worse, mounded up outside the barn, its rank, steaming heat enough to melt the snow around it.

Victor had to clean the pens out before school, clean them again before supper. "Got to keep them hogs healthy", the old man would say. "They all we got in the world." In spring, they would spread the winter's manure on the fields, hoping for rain to settle the nutrients down into the soil, but the stuff just dried up like the earth and the wind blew flecks of desiccated excrement into Victor's eyes and nose and mouth, where they moistened enough to let him taste the same foulness he was smelling.

Pigs were everything on the Whitehall farm: their fattening, their health, their breeding, and most of all their price on the hoof— which never seemed to rise no matter how much Victor's father planned and prayed and figured with a stubbed pencil on the back of an unpaid bill.

By the time he was ten, they paid off the last hired hand even though he was willing to work just for food and tobacco, and the pig shit became Victor's responsibility. He was big enough then to drive the flap-eared hogs from one pen to another, whacking them in the face with the old hickory cane when they went for his ankles. Then he'd shovel the turd-and-urine soaked straw into the wooden wheelbarrow and haul it outside.

The pigs were everything. The old man planted most of their sixty acres in fodder corn for the stock, but the long drought left the soil so worn out and dry that even in a good year—which was really just a not-so-bad year—the stalks barely stood above Victor's head, and he was never tall.

When the farm had been new, his mama put in apple and pear saplings, grafted so they would yield fruit early. But then the rains stopped coming and the trees stopped growing, so by the time Victor was fourteen—his mother long since run off with the fertilizer salesman from Tulsa—the orchard was three rows of dwarf trees, producing hard, sour fruits that went to the pigs. Sent to gather the miniature harvest, Victor would pretend he was a giant in a story, stomping through a forest looking for a village to smash.

When he was fifteen, he saw his father get beaten by the men from the bank who came to take the pigs and the farm, chasing the squealing hogs into a slat-sided Ford truck and piling their few sticks of furniture and their bedding on the road. Victor's old man threw himself against the little weed in round-lensed glasses who brought the piece of paper that said the bank now owned it all, but a beefy man in a fedora and sweat-stained suit grabbed Victor's father by the back of his collar and brought a leather-covered sap down hard. The first blow settled the issue; the second was unnecessary and it broke something inside the balding head so that always after the old man didn't walk quite the same, and couldn't remember well.

They ended up in a hobo jungle beside the tracks south of Tulsa. The old man met up with a rangy Texan named Red who had worked for them once, and the former hired hand showed them how to get along in the jungle.

Victor's father took to sitting around on the stumps and busted out old chairs by somebody's fire, cadging drinks of hooch that was brewed up from sugar and moldy potatoes. To get a drink, the old man would trade the food that Victor brought back from town, some of it begged, some stolen, rarely paid for by a day's chores for some kind-hearted woman or mean-spirited bastard who would work him ten hours for a day-old loaf and some dry beans.

One day he came back with a chunk of salt pork, the first meat he'd seen in longer than he could recall, determined that he was going to eat his share and make his father choke down his portion. But the old man was gone. He and Red had tried to lift whatever they could from a freight they'd caused to slow down by piling trash on the tracks. Railroad bulls jumped them while they were jimmying a boxcar's top hatch, kicked and clubbed them and ran them in to face the judge. Neither man came back and word was they'd be on the chain gang for six months.

Victor didn't see any point waiting. The road was safer at night than the jungle for boy who hadn't grown much, even one who kept a railroad spike ready to smash the head of any man who tried to take what was his, like the gap-toothed West Virginian with the coal dust flecked deep in the pores of his nose who thought he could help himself to their goods one time when the old man was drunk.

There was no point waiting for his father. The six-month sentence the judge handed down meant nothing once a man was in the grip of a chain gang boss; their labor was sold to whoever would pay, and as long as they could work they were money in the boss's pocket. Victor bundled up what little he had in a suitcase tied with a rope and set out for the oil fields around Enid. Guys said there was work there.

He caught a freight the first fifty miles or so, but when it pulled into a siding to wait for a passenger train to go through the bulls swept the cars clean. He hiked a half mile to a county road where he could put out his thumb. Traffic was scarce and he walked another couple of miles in the mid-day heat to where a ramshackle hay barn stood close enough to the road to throw some shade. In the afternoon a farmer in a Model A truck gave him a ride to a paved two-lane that ran to a town called Ephraim. The man let him have a drink of water and a couple of potatoes then ran him through to the far side of town. He warned Victor not to go into Ephraim or the sheriff would have him cutting weeds in leg irons.

The boy put another mile between him and the town. He settled in the shade of a peeled and faded billboard, only coming out when he heard a car.

Late in the afternoon, a Chevrolet coupe stopped, its paint a deep, lustrous blue with hardly a smear of dust. When Victor climbed in, the interior had a leathery smell that reminded him of a new-oiled harness, laid over by the scent of hair pomade from the man at the wheel.

"How far you want to go?" the man said. He was fat, in a cream-colored suit and tan and white wingtips, his pink jowls overhanging the collar of his shirt.

"Enid," Victor said. "Hear there's work there."

The man shifted up through the gears, a thick gold ring on the little finger of his hand flashing in the afternoon sun. When the Chev was in third gear, the hand came down and patted Victor's thigh, midway up from his knee. The boy felt its damp warmth through the thin cloth of his trousers. "I can take you a fair piece along the way," the man said.

He said little about himself: it seemed he sold what he called "the comforts of life" to people who hadn't been busted down by the Depression, the people who bought up land dirt cheap after the banks had repossessed it or counties had seized it for non-payment of taxes. "It's a hard world for the many, but a good life for the deserving few," he told Victor, his small eyes glinting in a wink and his gelatinous lips shaping a thickened smile.

He asked a lot of questions: where are your folks? any relatives in these parts? anybody looking out for you? The boy answered briefly. The man's hand came back to his thigh, moved higher, stayed a while. Victor reached for the suitcase he had placed on the floor of the car, edge-up between his legs, when he had got in. He laid the battered leather across his thighs and unroped it, reaching in to take out one of the potatoes the farmer had given him. He asked the man if he wanted a bite, but the salesman looked away in disdain. While his gaze was averted, Victor slipped his spike out of the suitcase and laid it on the seat beside his right leg, out of sight.

The sun was going down and they were on a narrow dirt road that seemed to go nowhere, although the man had called it a short cut. There were some trees up ahead, darkness growing beneath them, where a dry stream bed was culverted under the road. The salesman steered the Chev into the gloom and cut the engine. "How'd you like to make a buck?" he said.

The hobo jungle had taught Victor things he hadn't known about on a pig farm, like what happened between men and boys in state and county lock-ups. He'd heard that sometimes those relationships were negotiated, but mostly they were settled by force. He saw how the salesman looked at him, his eyes set among creases in a round, pale face. He'd seen that look in a hog pen.

He reached for the door handle but it rattled loose in his hand. "Busted," the fat man said, turning in the seat to face the boy. "You know, I keep meaning to get that fixed." The only other way out was the door against which his cloth covered back was now leaning.

"You better let me go," Victor said.

"You better think about that dollar." The man took the suitcase off the boy's lap and threw it into the back seat. He leisurely unbuckled his belt and began to unbutton his flies. "You turn out to be a good learner, might even earn yourself an extra quarter."

He put both hands on the waistband of his loosened pants and began to shrug them down, moving his fat buttocks to free the cloth. The boy turned and kneeled on the seat facing him, and when the man said, "Well, now..." Victor hit him in the temple with the chisel-like point of the spike, hit him hard the way he used to hit the pigs to drive them back.

The metal went in through the thin bone and Victor had to work it back and forth a couple of times to free it, then he hit the man again, this time on the top of his head, the edge of the spike cracking the bone. The man was making noises and moving his arms and legs, but he didn't seem to have much control over where his limbs were going. Victor hit him again in the same spot, blood gushing out over the greasy hair, then a third time that went through bone and deep into softness. The man stopped making noises, slumping forward, and now the high, sharp stink of excrement overcame the scent of hair oil and car leather.

Victor reached behind the dead man's back, found the door handle and yanked it down. The inert form fell backward through the opening, into the darkness and down a slope and was gone, only the smell remaining. Victor shut the door and settled himself in the driver's seat. He had driven his father's old truck before they'd had to sell it. He got the engine going again and found that the gears were not that different from what he knew. He put the car back on the road and drove away, spewing a plume of dust that blocked his view of what was behind him.

A mile on, he realized that he should have taken the man's wallet and thought about going back—but he didn't want to smell that stink ever again. He found a road that led south and drove a long way. Then the Chev's lighted dials told him that it was low on fuel. He came to a railroad crossing and drove another mile, then walked back and waited. At dawn a milk train came by and he ran beside it, his suitcase tight under his arm, and caught the steel ladder at one end of a flatbed car. He tucked himself behind some milk cans and rode until the train slowed near a dairy farm, then he jumped clear and found a bush to sleep under.

It was past noon when he woke. He found the railroad spike in his jacket pocket, sticky with blood and stuff that didn't look much different from pig brains. He cleaned it with grass and put it in his hip pocket, then ate the last of his potato as he walked south. Later on he got a ride with a man who was delivering tools to an oil camp and learned that the best way to get work was not to approach a camp boss and ask for wages, but to ask the camp cook to take him on for food and a place to sleep. "Costs nothing to feed a cook-tent flunky on scraps while you're doing half the cook's work, and the shit half at that," the man said.

Victor got hired on as a cook's helper in the third drilling camp he found, working for food and a place at the back of the kitchen tent. The cook drove him like a hired mule, but he'd worked harder for less and now he started to fill out. It was April when he walked into the camp, just as the first drill frame was going up; by the end of June he was ten pounds heavier, all of it muscle from lifting tubs of potatoes and dishwater. The men left him alone, and after a couple of weeks, he stopped carrying the railroad spike in his back pocket. He pushed it down into the hard dirt behind the cook tent and put a rock over it.

Mitch Halloran was the drill boss, a skinny wildcatter with thinning hair and a Clark Gable mustache. This was a spec hole and the drilling was paid for partially on Halloran's nickel but mostly on the bank's. If he came up dry, there'd be no more draw for the men's wages and everything in the camp, from the derrick and drill bits to the galvanized tub where Victor stooped to wash tin plates and spoons, would be seized and sold.

Like many wildcatters, Halloran believed in luck and looked for omens, so when it happened that the well came in with a gusher just as Victor Whitehall was bringing him coffee and biscuits, he took it as a sign. As the boy turned to go back to the cook tent, Halloran said, "Hold it. What's your name, kid?"

"Victor."

The boss nodded. "Good name." He wiped some of the oil from his hands and reached for a biscuit. "Can you read and write?"

"Yes, sir."

"Can you figure?"

"My pa taught me after I stopped going to school."

"What's eight times seven?"

Victor didn't hesitate. "Fifty-six, sir."

"How much am I paying you?"

"Nothing. Just meals and a place to sleep."

"Not any more. Here on in, it's a dollar a day plus your keep. You'll be my helper."

"Yes, sir."

"Go get cleaned up and tell cookie he has to do his own goddamn work from now on. Then get back here."

• • •

Victor Whitehall stayed with Mitch Halloran for seven years, learning everything there was to know about drilling for oil. The war came and went, but Victor didn't go into the services; the business of fueling destroyers, tanks and bombers took precedence. It turned out he was a fast learner with a natural gift for the hard sciences of chemistry and geology, although his learning was entirely focused on the practicalities of finding oil and getting it out of the ground.

He also turned out to be more than lucky for Halloran Exploration Company. He had a talent for knowing where the liquid gold would be found; Victor could stand on a piece of ground and know if there was oil half a mile below his feet. It was as if he could smell it through the earth.

"I heard of guys like you," Halloran said. "Dowsers, they call them. But I never really believed it."

In time, they might have become true friends, but in 1948, Mitch Halloran died under the wheels of a rig truck that backed over him on an east Texas drill site. Relatives sold the company to a Dallas consortium. Victor had no stake in the business; he'd just been an employee. But at twenty-four he was a seasoned hand in the oil exploration business with a strong reputation as a reliable finder of fresh reserves. He set up as a lease agent, finding sites with good potential on private and public lands and negotiating for companies looking to drill. He took commissions instead of fees so his talent for finding underground riches soon earned him enough to buy his own rigs and hire crews. Victor Whitehall did well, and then he did very well.

At thirty he was a multi-millionaire in an age when top executives were earning twenty thousand a year. He owned producing fields in the US, in Canada and in Venezuela that poured cash into Whitehall Holdings, Inc., cash that he turned into assets, buying companies and fitting them into a growing empire. He had a nose for companies that were undercapitalized, where an infusion of money and a ruthless management style would transform pokey little enterprises into going concerns.

At forty-three, he was worth a billion. At fifty, it was two billion and still rising. He had his own office tower in Manhattan, close by Wall Street, where he could usually sniff out an acquirable bargain before other market movers even knew there was blood in the air. From his top-floor suite he looked out to the edge of the world. His office was spacious but spartan, and on a credenza behind his wide desk was a rusty railroad spike mounted on a piece of hardwood. Whitehall used it as a gavel when he chaired meetings.

Thirty years after he left the hobo jungle he thought to find out what had happened to his father. It turned out that the old man had died of heat stroke while chopping weeds on the Tulsa chain gang. Whitehall received the news without comment.

He rarely drank and never much, but he kept a few bottles in a sideboard for visitors, because oil and liquor have always mixed. After he heard about his father, he sat while the afternoon turned to dusk, drinking whatever there was. At six, his assistant came in and asked if he wanted to be driven home.

Whitehall told him, "In this world, you can either be a pig or you can be a chicken. It's not a good thing to be a pig. But it's a godawful thing to be a chicken."

• • •

At seventy-eight years old, Victor Whitehall looked no more than sixty. His skin was pink and his eyes were sharp and he had put on more than enough flesh to bury forever the skinny boy who had shoveled hog manure and seen his daddy beaten into the dust. He came into the large room adjacent to his office on Friday morning to find his key staff ranged around the oblong slab of polished variegated marble that was the Whitehall Holdings conference table. He sat in the middle of one long side, rapped a block of wood with his railroad spike and said, "Let's hear reports."

One by one his senior executives reported on their areas of responsibility, while their employer nodded or asked brief follow-up questions. It was a smooth process, well honed over years of operations, and took less than a half hour to complete. Then Whitehall fixed his gaze on the silver-haired man in an understated pinstripe who sat directly across the center of the table from him. Arthur Pennock returned the stare with an expression of polite attention that did not fool Victor Whitehall. There was an odor of fear beneath the corporate lawyer's expensive aftershave.

"What more do we know about Flynnt?" Whitehall asked.

Pennock cleared his throat, not quite inaudibly, and said, "There's another placement of stock in the works. Approximately two hundred million's worth. Yukio Ishihara is the purchaser."

"And is that covered?"

"Yes, sir. Ishihara will sell the shares on to us at a twelve per cent premium."

Whitehall's bristling eyebrows folded down, half obscuring his eyes. "Twelve? That's a pretty good return for holding a stock less than twenty-four hours."

"Ishihara's being a hard ass," Pennock said. "He's figured out we want to make a move on Flynnt, so he's screwing us for the extra two per."

Whitehall made a sound deep in his throat then moved on. "All, right, fuck the two per cent. We'll get it back down the road when we've got something the Jap wants. What I really want to know is if we're picking up any noise—I mean anything—about what Terry Flynnt's up to. Why is he putting together this pool of cash?"

Pennock looked as if only years of practice were preventing him from squirming under his employer's gaze. "We don't know anything more than we knew last week. They've finished building whatever they were building on his island, still looks like some kind of research unit. One of our watchers said they flew in a man and a woman the other day from Miami."

"Who were they?"

"The woman appears to be Hilary Cartiere, remember her? The guy we don't know yet. He's nobody in business, I mean nobody of size."

Whitehall thought about it. "Friends of the racing driver and the liberal clothes horse?"

Pennock nodded. "It's what I'm thinking. Flynnt wasn't there when they arrived. We know he was still on his yacht."

"Check it anyway." Whitehall leaned his forearms on the cold stone. "Something's happening with Flynnt. There's weakness there, I can smell it."

"We need someone on the inside," Pennock said.

Whitehall turned to his chief of security, an ex-CIA assistant director named Fletcher. "Well?"

Fletcher affected tweeds and a mid-Atlantic accent. "Isaac Dumoulin knows what he's doing," he said. "We send them in, he turns them around, kicks their arses out the door."

"Can we turn somebody who's already in?" Whitehall said.

"Not so far. Flynnt pays well and Dumoulin terrifies even better."

"This is not good enough."

Fletcher opened his mouth, then decided it was better to close it.

"What?" Whitehall said.

"I have one idea," Fletcher said.

"Say it."

"There's a fellow we've used down there on a couple of 'assignments,'" he said, giving an emphasis to the word that meant that the work had involved somebody's blood and pain, and probably worse. "Name's Larkin. Former British SBS—like Navy Seals."

"I know what the Special Boat Service is," Whitehall said.

"I thought we could send him in to look around the island and the boat. He's smart enough to know good information if he comes across it and he's good enough to maybe get in and out through Dumoulin's security."

"What's the downside?"

"He won't let himself get caught."

Whitehall shrugged. "That's the way it should be."

"No, it's more than that. He spent two months in a Yemeni jail. If he thinks he's going to go in the bag, he'll resist by all means."

"He'll kill some of Flynnt's people. We can live with that."

Fletcher shook his head. "But if he's in Flynnt's office and Flynnt comes in... that's going to be it for Flynnt."

Whitehall drew a long breath that made his bulk swell even larger, then let it go. "We're not ready for that yet."

"Then all we can do is keep digging for a weak spot," Fletcher said.

"Then dig hard," Whitehall said. "I know we can take this one. Now go and get it for me."

He rapped the wood with the stained spike. He didn't have to say, "or else."

Chapter 10

Carras awoke to the sensation of movement, but none of it was his. His arms and legs were tightly bound, his ankles connected to his wrists so that he lay on his side in a fetal position. There was something across his mouth—tape, he thought. He struggled to move his limbs but found that Isaac's competence extended to the hog-tying of surgeons.

He saw only darkness, but the hiss of tires on asphalt told him he was in the trunk of a car. He thought about stories of kidnap victims who worked out where they were held by remembering sound cues heard along the route. He listened, but no handy jackhammers or circus calliopes made auditory landmarks. Besides, he had a pretty good idea where he was being taken, and his deduction was confirmed when the car stopped and Isaac and Maigrot opened the trunk.

They were in a hangar, right next to Flynnt's jet. There was nobody else in sight. Isaac reached in and scooped Carras up like a B-movie monster carrying off the helpless heroine, and in less than a minute the three of them were in a bedroom in the rear of the luxury jet. Isaac laid the doctor on the bed and tucked a thermal blanket tight around his already bound limbs. Then he pulled the tape away from Carras's mouth. It hurt just as much as Carras had always suspected it would.

"You won't get away with this," he said. It was a cliché but he meant it all the same.

"Sure we will," Isaac said. "Crew's been told I'm sleeping in here and they're not to bother me." He looked beyond the head of the bed and said, "Come on, let's go."

Maigrot was up there somewhere. Carras couldn't turn his head far enough to see him, but he could hear noises. It sounded like a cellophane wrapped package being opened.

"What are you going to do?" Carras said.

Isaac didn't answer. He was still looking at Maigrot beyond the head of the bed and for the first time Carras saw irritation reshape his ordinarily impassive features. Finally he said, "Give me the damn thing."

Maigrot's voice had a tremor in it. "This is bad, Isaac."

"I'm not going to argue with you, Leonard. Some things have to be done. Legal, illegal, doesn't come into it. Want to, don't want to, doesn't matter. This is necessary."

"Kidnaping is a federal crime," Maigrot said.

"You already did the crime," Isaac said, "when you helped put him in the car. It's too late for forgive and forget." He looked down at Carras. "We let you go, you going to let bygones be bygones?"

Carras said, "Maybe."

Isaac laughed. "Man, you are a cool one," he said.

"What are you going to do with me?" Carras asked again.

"Change your mind," Isaac said. He reached toward Maigrot and his hand came back holding a hypodermic needle.

A chill went through Carras. He pulled against the bonds. "What's in that?"

"Just to quiet you down," Isaac said.

The injection stung Carras's shoulder like a wasp that had taken a personal dislike. But the pain faded almost instantly as the drug cut in. Something heavy, Carras thought, as the glow began to spread: an opiate, maybe demerol. He settled back into the bed. The mattress was softer, warmer.

"There you go," Isaac said. He removed the blanket and cut the cords around Carras's ankles and wrists. The doctor stretched, took a long slow breath that felt like a distillation of summer afternoons and slid down into an easy gentleness that enfolded him like God's hand, warm and safe and all around. He heard Isaac saying to Maigrot, "Get the car detailed..." then he was gone.

He remembered only moments from the next several hours, and some of the moments probably never happened. Certainly, Beth and Costas didn't come and sit with him and talk about things that he could never quite focus on; even as the words formed in his mind they fluttered away, dissolving as they drifted off. He was pretty sure he remembered night and the sound of surf and a breeze that smelled of the sea. Maigrot and Isaac were holding him between them, his feet taking steps he couldn't feel, though he could see the wood of a wharf beneath them. Then another brief pricking at his shoulder and it all went away again.

· · ·

Something rough was against his cheek. He felt it catch the stubble of his beard when he stirred. There was a smell, like fruit rotting in damp earth. Almost, he fell back into the soft dream, but the warm hand of God no longer held him.

He opened eyes that were gummed from too long a sleep, his corneas covered by a film that hazed his vision. He blinked and it cleared. Now he was looking at rough wood, horizontal planks of some rough lumber, knotted and splintery: a wall, only inches away. He was lying on his side on a filthy burlap sack, facing the wall of a wooden shack. His hand came up to rub his face and he found that he was unbound.

He heard a shriek, close by. Carras rolled onto his back, hands out to fend off. The light in the windowless shack was dim, only a faint glow leaking in from around the loosely fitted door. Something was between him and the light, something dark and making a lot of high-pitched noise. At first he couldn't get his eyes to focus on it, then he rubbed them and the shape resolved itself into a small black boy in tattered shorts, skinny-armed but with a protruding belly, his eyes big, round and white as he hammered with tiny fists against the door and shouted something that sounded like *leeravy*.

It was when the child added another word—it sounded like *mess-yeh*—that it fell into place for Carras. The boy was crying for the attention of someone beyond the locked door, and language he was speaking was *Kreyol*, the creole of French and African languages that was spoken only in the island nation of Haiti.

"*Mesye!*" the boy shrieked again. "*Li reveye! Li reveye!*" Mister! He's waking up! Whoever "Mister" was, he'd left the child in the shed to be a human motion detector and alarm.

Carras sat up, felt the space around him spin as blood briefly fled his brain. He was weak. He hadn't eaten in a long time, at least a day and probably more while they had drugged and transported him two thousand miles. To Haiti.

That was the first mistake he'd caught Flynnt's people making. This time they hadn't done their research well enough, or they would have known that even though it wasn't on his curriculum vitae Carras had been to Haiti. Back in the seventies all Yale surgeons-in-training served a three-month rotation at the Albert Schweitzer Hospital in Haiti's back of nowhere.

His head was clearing now, the focused mind finding something to lock onto. He was frightened, but he focused on the fact that Flynnt had made a mistake. The billionaire would want his captive to be disoriented, waking up in some primitive hell-hole, not knowing where he was, people shouting in a language he didn't understand. Disorientation would bring fear and fear would make Carras vulnerable. *But I know something they think I don't know,* Carras thought. It was a small edge but the only one he had.

There was a rattle of a chain then the door opened to let the boy out. The shack was lit by a glare of tropical light that was instantly darkened by a wide-shouldered man who filled the narrow entry. He stepped inside and Carras saw that he was clothed in sweat-stained cotton pants and shirt, a broad brimmed straw hat pulled low over his forehead and a faded red bandana around his neck. His skin was lighter than Isaac's, the color of coffee with plenty of cream. The expression he showed Carras was not friendly.

In one hand he held a bundle of cloth, and this he now threw to the earthen floor. Carras looked down and realized he was naked. He was to wear the rags the man had tossed him: a pair of greasy shorts and a stained sleeveless shirt with a ripped collar. The man's other hand held a pair of straw sandals with soles cut from a tire.

Carras put on the rags while the man watched. The doorway darkened again and a woman came in, light skinned and grossly pregnant, carrying a plastic jug of water and something wrapped in large leaves. She bent to set the things down in front of the prisoner, grunting as she rose. Carras saw a look of concern break through the man's stern expression. He filed the information away.

With the woman gone, the man indicated the bundle of leaves. *Mange ca,* he growled. *Puis travail.* Eat that, then work, Carras translated. That was not the Haitian *patois,* but basic French. That meant the man was probably the *patron,* the boss or overseer of whatever this place was.

Carras gave no indication he understood the French, but opened up the bundle. It was cold rice and beans wrapped in banana leaf. The water in the jug looked clean, but Carras knew it would harbor a flourishing population of bugs and floaters. He might still be resistant to some of them, courtesy of his seasoning twenty-three years before when his stint at the Schweitzer had given him two serious fevers and a week of mild dysentery.

He ate and drank while the man watched him. When he was finished, he said, because it would be expected of him, "Who are you? What is this place?"

"*Tais toi*", said the man—shut up—and gestured with a thumb for Carras to get up and follow him. It was not yet mid-morning, judging by the height of the sun, but the heat slapped against Carras's head and shoulders like noon on the hottest day New Haven ever knew. Sweat beaded instantly on his head and the back of his neck, and he felt a trickle down his side.

The cream-colored man tapped his chest. "*Je m'appelles Falardeau,*" he said, then tapped again. "*Falardeau, compris?*"

"Falardeau," Carras said. He touched his own chest. "Carras," he said.

Falardeau said something that Carras didn't catch, but the look on his face indicated that he had used whatever the local expression was for who gives a rat's ass? Then he said, "*Tu fais c'que je dis, ou...*" and raised a fist that displayed well scarred knuckles. You do what I tell you, or you can meet my strongest argument.

Carras put up both hands in the universal gesture that said Falardeau was the boss. He wasn't going to fight when he was sure to lose. The only thing he wanted out of this place was out of this place, and he wouldn't get that by taking a beating in his first half hour.

They were in a Haitian village street, a muddy track that straggled between cinder block houses and shacks cobbled together from scrap lumber and tar paper. They were most of the way up a broad, bare hill, covered by thin yellow grass. The commercial timber that had once grown here had been logged off for sale and the remaining "weed" trees had been gleaned for firewood. Around them were more stripped hills, but down in the bottoms between them were banana groves, the big funny looking trees that grew all over Haiti, producing cheap fruit for America's air-conditioned supermarkets.

The village was small, no more than forty homes, only one of them substantial enough—red-brick walls and corrugated steel roof—to be called a house. Carras guessed that would be Falardeau's. It was the highest set dwelling on the hill, and as he looked Carras saw the pregnant woman come out of its open doorway to throw a bucket of dirty liquid out into the bushes. She stopped, one hand to the small of her back. Again, Carras saw Falardeau's eyes go to her, dragging a worried look across his face.

Then the man came back to Carras. "*Allons-y,*" he said, and Carras didn't need to translate. The hand on his shoulder, turning him and pushing him toward a battered flat bed truck, told him that Falardeau had said, "Let's go."

Carras climbed onto the back. Falardeau got into the driver's seat and the gears clashed as the truck bounced down the rutted track toward the base of the hill. They went about a mile, Carras remembering the horrendous orthopedic injuries that used to come into the Schweitzer Hospital, when one of these Haitian *camions*, packed with passengers for whom it was the only transportation, would turn over on a so-called road on a hill like this. He stood and held on to a bar of steel that had been welded over the roof of the cab, the vehicle's sole concession to safety.

At the bottom of the slope the track was less prone to erosion during the torrents of rain that regularly sluiced the denuded Haitian hills. It leveled and smoothed out enough to be called a road, and they followed it for over a mile, close-packed banana trees on either side. Then Falardeau took them around a curve and the foliage dropped back on either side to reveal another kind of crop: tall, light colored stalks, leafy at the top, like bamboo but not bamboo. Sugar cane, Carras said to himself.

When he'd been at the Schweitzer hospital, sugar cane had been the big crop, both here and in the neighboring Dominican Republic, which shared the island of Hispaniola with Haiti. But the post-Duvalier government privatized the state-owned sugar mills just as international sugar prices crashed. The owners found it cheaper to import sugar made from sugar beets and use the former cane lands for bananas. Now just about the only cane sugar grown here was intended for local rum distillers. The old days were gone when cane fields ran for miles in all directions, but when the truck stopped there was enough cane in front of Carras to keep a handful of cutters in steady work.

There were six men, all skinny and very black, dressed much the way Carras was. The little boy who had sounded the alarm was also there, hanging back behind the adults. Carras guessed that his job after alerting Falardeau the overseer was to run down to the cane cutters and get them ready for the next scene in the drama. He had no doubt that something had been set up here, just as the meeting with Hilary and the bike race with Flynnt had been carefully arranged to manipulate him.

In this scene, he was supposed to be frightened and confused, having been plucked from his comfortable North American milieu and plunked down in a third world pest-hole. But he wasn't too frightened; Flynnt wouldn't want him killed or injured, because the end of the game as the billionaire saw it was to have Athan Carras on his feet in an operating theater, performing the transplant on his son Philip. But the heart would have come dripping from the chest of someone like the men standing in this cane field, perhaps a man who was selling his life—all at once, instead of day by day over a lifetime shortened by grinding poverty—so that his family might move out of this kind of hell.

That's not going to happen, Carras told himself. He was frightened—any sane man in his situation would be—but he wasn't confused at all. He knew where he was and he had a good idea of what would come next. *Travail*, Falardeau had said, and brought him to a cane field. They would make him work, try to make him think he was going to be worked to death, but the real goal was to break him down, break his spirit, so that when Isaac or Maigrot showed up in a week or so—it couldn't be too long; Philip didn't have too long—he'd be begging them to let him do the operation, anything to get out of the cane fields.

All right, he thought, *on with the show*. He put on a suitably apprehensive expression as Falardeau brought from the camion's cab a wide-bladed implement like a butcher's cleaver, except the blade was narrower at the handle and wider at its squared off end. This he held out to Carras with one hand, but the other hand offered a pair of soft leather gloves.

Carras took the three items and when Falardeau said, *"Met les gants,"* accompanying the words with appropriate gestures, the doctor tucked the knife between arm and ribs and pulled the supple leather over his hands.

"Bon," said the overseer and gestured to one of the crew, an older man with a tight cap of gray hair and sinewy arms in which veins clearly snaked their way across thin hard muscles. Carras remembered that fat people were a rare sight in Haitian villages—usually they were policemen or businessmen just passing through. Carras himself had lost twenty-five pounds in his three month sojourn, dropping from a lean 175 to a gaunt 150.

The man came over and took Carras's knife. He moved to the standing wall of cane, each stem almost twice a tall man's height and thick as a baseball bat. The man stooped and crooked his arm around a bundle of cane, pulled it toward him so it bent away from the rest of the crop, then swung the big knife into the stems close to the ground. The stained steel bit into the cane, but did not go through the entire bundle. The man worked the blade out then swung again, then gave the bundled canes another, final cut which separated them from their roots. He let the tall stalks fall to the ground then, still stooped, he moved a couple of feet down the stand, scooped another bundle and repeated the process. He stood up and handed the knife back to Carras.

Falardeau waved a hand toward the cane and said, *"Et maint'nant, c'est …
toi."* Now it's your turn.

Carras looked at the cane then back to the overseer. He shook his head. "No."

Falardeau let his eyebrows rise about half their full range, held them there for a few seconds then said, "No?"

"No," Carras said. They'd be suspicious if he gave in too quickly.

The overseer shrugged and went back to the cab of the camion, reached in again and came out with two more objects. One was a coiled whip of braided hide. The other was a submachine gun. He hung the weapon's strap over his shoulder and tossed the whip to the man with gray hair.

Then Falardeau pointed the machine pistol at Carras and ostentatiously drew back the bolt. The click was loud.

"Ti-Jean," he said. That would be the gray haired one's name, Carras thought, because now the man uncoiled the whip with a flick of his wrist, laying the length of leather among the stubble of cut cane.

Carras looked at Falardeau. The man had pulled his lower lip over his bottom teeth and now his free hand came out in a gesture that said, it's up to you, while the gun muzzle stayed pointed at the doctor's midriff.

The silence stretched through seconds, then Falardeau said to Ti-Jean, *"Pyes selman."*

Carras knew what it meant in creole: legs only. "Okay," he said. "*Je travail.*" I work. He deliberately mispronounced both words. He didn't want to give anything away.

"*Tu comprends le français?*" the overseer said.

Carras showed his gloved thumb and index finger, a half inch apart. "*Un peu,*" he said, again Americanizing the foreign vowels.

Falardeau squinted one eye. "*Pale kreyol?*" he said, thickening his Haitian accent.

Carras put on a puzzled look. "*Par le crayon?*" he said, and mimed writing on the palm of one hand. The overseer had asked him if he spoke creole, and he had responded as if the man had said, "with a pencil."

Falardeau grunted. "*N'importe,*" he said. Never mind. "*Travail, comprends?*"

Carras looked at the gun and the man with the whip, "*Je comprends,*" he said. He went to where Ti-Jean had cut two bundles, bent and pulled some cane toward him and slashed down with the knife. The black man had cut through his first stook of cane with two cuts and a finisher. Carras's first effort took five strokes before he could let the canes fall free beside him. The last cut had barely missed his foot.

He straightened and saw that the other cutters were watching with bemused expressions. Ti-Jean handed the whip to the little boy and took Carras's knife. He stooped and pulled some cane, then made a show of cutting down at an angle, nodding his head to indicate that this was the right way. Then he mimed cutting horizontally, level to the ground and shook his head, showing the blade passing through its arc and hitting his ankles. He handed the knife back.

"Got it," Carras said. He was relieved. Clearly, they didn't want him hurt, just hurting. He pulled another bundle of cane toward him and struck down with the blade. The others watched to see that he was doing it right then they all went back to work, Ti-Jean surrendering the whip and taking up a cane knife. Falardeau sat in the open door of the truck, his feet on the step-up and the machine pistol across his knees.

The work was hard. Carras was in good shape; he had to be—surgery involves hours of standing bent over a table. Muscles that aren't well toned won't take the strain. He worked out on exercise machines at least three times a week, and rode his bike or jogged almost every day. But this was something else. He'd heard of stoop labor, but had never thought of what it really meant to work crooked over, with a monotonous output of muscle power: pull, chop, chop, chop again, sweat running in his eyes, trickling down his chest and soaking the waistband of his shorts.

After ten minutes his right forearm had begun to swell, as if he were wrist-curling a dumbbell. Blood flow was blocked by the swollen tissue and

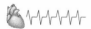

the arm started to ache. The long muscles in the backs of his thighs also began to complain, so he stopped and stood upright to stretch. Immediately, pains like thin bladed knives sliced through his lower back. He flexed his glutes and heard lumbar vertebrae crack like knuckles as they repositioned themselves.

Holy shit, he thought, if a few minutes make me hurt this bad, how'm I going to put up with a day of it?

Because it would have to be at least a day before he could run. But run he would. Maybe get down to the coast that was seldom far away in Haiti, steal a boat, get the hell out of here. Either along the coast to the Dominican Republic and the US embassy, or out into the Caribbean and flag down the first decent sized craft that came along. Or offer a local fisherman a thousand dollars to land him in Florida.

All he needed to know was the way to the coast, and then wait for the first unguarded moment—maybe dig his way out of that hut they'd kept him in—and run for it.

"*Eh, au travail!*" Falardeau called from the truck, lifting the gun for emphasis. Carras went back to work, gritting his teeth against the pains in his back and thighs. He wondered how much of this he could endure, then realized that was precisely the thought Flynnt wanted him to be having at this moment. *Bastard!* he thought. *We'll see.*

It was going to be about more than just escaping, a lot more. First would come beating Flynnt at his game; then would come revenge. He wasn't a third world field hand; he was a prominent member of the American medical profession—one of the best doctors in America—and he would bring the law down on Terry Flynnt. Kidnapping, extortion, assault, unlawful confinement. While he pulled and cut, he itemized the charges. Administering a noxious substance, wasn't that an offense? He remembered the opiate flooding through his system. He wouldn't mind some of the analgesic effect right now.

The sweat was coming off him in sheets, the heat of the tropical mid-day rising to its worst. The parched soil threw the heat back in his face so that he was being baked from above and below. He straightened, felt the knives even worse now, and wiped his face with the hem of his shirt.

He looked at Falardeau and said, "*Boire, besoin de boire.*" Drink, need to drink, again mispronouncing the French.

The overseer smiled, but it wasn't pleasant. "*Ça fait chaud, non?*" Hot enough for you?

Carras swallowed though there was no moisture in his mouth now. "*Boire,*" he said, then made it seem that he was hunting for the words, "*ou mort.*" Drink or death.

Falardeau shrugged and looked up at the sun, but after letting it ride for a moment, he reached behind him and brought out a plastic bottle and tossed it to Carras. "*Pas trop,*" he said. Not too much.

Carras uncapped the bottle and drank a little of the tepid water, then a little more. He put the mouth of the container to his lips again, but Falardeau said, "*Assez.*" Enough.

Carras put the bottle down, but did not immediately go back to work. "*Chapeau,*" he said, pointing to his head. He needed a hat. He pointed to the sun. "*Le sol.*"

There was only one hat in sight, and it was on Falardeau's head. He touched it and said, "*Non.*"

"*Mort,*" said Carras, tapping his chest.

Falardeau shrugged, but he didn't order Carras back to work. Instead he called over the little boy and said something to him. The child ran off but was back moments later with two large banana leaves. Falardeau took these and quickly twisted and folded, producing a hat such as Robinson Crusoe might have worn before he killed and skinned his first wild goat. "*Voilá...,*" he said and sent the child to bring it to Carras.

The boy held it out at arm's length, clearly not wanting to get any closer than he had to. Carras took the thing, said, "*Merci,*" and put it on his head. He saw Falardeau laughing and knew he must look ridiculous—that was how they wanted him to look and feel. He made sure that the expression on his face was suitably woeful and went back to the agonizing work.

It had been another test. The water and the hat said that his well-being was important. They could have let him overheat before they answered his physical needs. He thought about it as he pulled and cut and moved on, rising above the pain to focus his mind, just as he would have done near the end of a long operation, when his calf muscles would be aching from six or seven hours of standing. They would not kill him, nor would they cause him more than superficial harm—the whip across his legs, but no risk of fatal heatstroke. He noticed he was the only cutter wearing gloves: they'd have been warned not to damage his hands.

So if he ran, they would chase him but not shoot at him. The pursuit would be dedicated, but they would not bring out dogs that might rip the wrong part of him, say his precious hands, because that would leave him unable to operate. Falardeau would pretend to have the power of life and death over him, but underneath his pose of ruthless authority, the overseer would be worrying about keeping his captive alive and whole.

Time went by. Between the monotony of the labor and the concentration of his thoughts, Carras hardly noticed. But then Ti-Jean was beside him, touching his shoulder. Carras turned and stood erect, the back pain much worse this time, and followed the black man to the truck, where Falardeau was handing out packages of leaf-wrapped food from a tattered basket. He gave one to his prisoner with a sarcastic, "*Bon appetit.*"

The other men trooped across the track to the banana fields and sat down

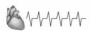

in the shade. Carras went with them, but sat a little apart. Falardeau followed, the child at his heels, and sat where he could watch the prisoner. He put the machine pistol on the ground beside him, in easy reach, and opened his own parcel, which seemed to be the same as what Carras and the others had.

It was rice again, but with bits of vegetable and peppers instead of beans. There was also a small fish, cooked with head and tail still on. It had an oily taste, but after the work Carras had a good appetite. He had brought his bottle of water to drink from, but the cutters had a larger container, a plastic jug that would hold at least a gallon, and this they were passing around. By the time it was half gone, the men's mood seemed to have improved and Carras deduced that it must contain some home-made brew, maybe even watered rum from the cane they were cutting.

He remembered from his time in Haiti that the mid-day siesta was an institution here. If they emptied the jug and fell asleep, an opportunity for escape could arise. He could drive the truck, maybe to some place where there was a phone. Then a call to the US embassy and... But he saw that Falardeau wasn't drinking, though the overseer watched the jug go around with unconcealed regret. And when the men stretched themselves on the ground to sleep, Falardeau remained alert. He dragged the gun onto his lap, leaned his back against a banana tree's leafy trunk and kept his eyes on Carras.

The prisoner finished the meal, licking the last grains of rice from the leaves and his fingers, and looked about him. He put on a suitably nervous expression and said, "*Monsieur, où sommes nous?*"

Falardeau laughed a short laugh. "*L'arriere d'enfer,*" he said. The back end of hell.

Carras looked around at the banana trees and the men sleeping on the ground. "*C'est Afrique?*" he said.

The overseer laughed again. "*Bien sur,*" he said. "*L'Afrique.*" You bet we're in Africa.

Carras managed a small shudder. "*Que passez ... moi?*" It was mangled French for what will happen to me?

"*Tu attends, tu apprends.*" Wait and see. "*Alors, dormes-toi.*"

Having assured Falardeau that he did not know where they were and was worried about it, Carras did as he was told, stretching himself out in the shade and laying his head on his arm. His back and legs ached but he fell asleep within moments. Still, it seemed like no time before Falardeau's booted toe prodded his ribs. "*Travail,*" the overseer said.

The afternoon was worse than the morning. Carras's muscles had stiffened while he slept and the first few minutes of cane cutting were an unparalleled agony. Then his body warmed to the exertion—the sun helped too—and the pain receded to an ache that was still bad but bearable. His mind returned to the question of escape. He wondered what happened to the truck's keys at night. He would watch to see what Falardeau did with them when they went back up the dirt track.

The cane field was alive with insects, things that buzzed in the ear, some of them settling to bite and draw blood. He swatted at them, thinking about malaria and the fevers he'd contracted when he had been in Haiti before, but there was no use worrying. He could enlist some of the world's best in tropical medicine once he got out of here. But getting out had to come first.

He fell into a kind of waking doze, the pain and exertion driving him out of ordinary consciousness. After a while, he heard a louder buzzing in his ear and waved a hand to shoo the insect away. But the sound did not change, except to grow louder. He was puzzled until he understood that he was hearing the distant engine of a light plane, and not too distant. He stood and stretched. The aircraft, a single-engined type, was low over the hills to the north.

He immediately bent back to his work, but his ears kept the sound of the plane in the forefront of his mind. He heard its drone, fading in and out. But the plane had been very low, and now the sound abruptly stopped. It must have gone behind a hill. And if it went behind a hill, it either crashed, he thought, or it landed.

He stretched and looked north again, but there was no distant boom, no rising plume of smoke. The plane had gone down the way it was supposed to, and that meant there was an airport—at least an airstrip—not many miles away. He couldn't fly a plane, but he could hire or bribe someone to take him up and out of here. Now all he needed was the opportunity to get there.

They didn't work as late as Carras feared they might. Well short of evening, his legs began to tremble and his cuts with the cane knife became too weak to be effective. Just when he felt that a complete collapse was not far off, Falardeau had the men erect the wooden sides of the flat bed truck. The overseer drove it along the lanes of cut cane and they loaded the crop aboard then climbed on themselves. Carras had to be pulled aboard by Ti-Jean and one of the younger men. He sprawled on the hard stems while white fire shot through his lower back and thighs with every bounce and sway of the camion. The Haitians spoke to each other in relaxed voices and laughed over a joke that one of them made.

To Carras, they didn't look or sound like men who'd done a hard day of stoop labor, even allowing for a lifetime's practice. He followed the thought and remembered that when he had arrived, well into the morning, there had been no cut cane on the ground. It's all a show, he told himself, all part of the set-up. They must figure he would endure no more than a couple or three days before surrendering, and then Falardeau and the men would go back to working the banana crop.

Okay, he thought, *I'm the victim here. I'll play the victim. Let them see what they expect to see.* That would be the screen behind which he would watch for an opportunity, then emerge to seize it.

He didn't have to play-act when he arrived back at the village. He slid down the pile of cane and off the back of the truck with a heartfelt groan. Falardeau and Ti-Jean half-carried him to the storage hut. He sank onto the pile of ill-smelling sacking with relief.

"*On t'emenera … manger,*" Falardeau said. Someone would bring him food. Then he shut the door and Carras heard a latch drop into place. For several minutes, he lay on the coarse cloth, then he rolled onto his stomach and began massaging the strained muscles of his lower back, working some circulation through them before they stiffened beyond hope. As he rubbed and stretched, he made a careful examination of his prison.

He thought it might have been a storage site for dry goods, sacks of grain, maybe. The walls were of thick horizontal planks, tight against each other and nailed onto an internal structure of two-by-four studs. There was a strong frame of doubled two-by-fours that formed the door jamb and lintel and the roof was more planks with shingle nails coming through. The floor was earth, packed hard as concrete.

Carras rolled over and sat up, rubbed his thighs and calves. After dark he would test all the planks, but he had no real hope of finding a loose one. He could get out of here if he had some metal tool to cut the wood or dig the earth, but as long as he had only his fingernails and teeth, he'd be staying.

A cane knife would be ideal, but they had taken his from him before he was hauled onto the truck. Even if he could lay his hands on a spare, he doubted he could hide it under his skimpy clothing. He'd have to watch for something just lying around, a nail or a hunk of scrap iron, some piece of junk that meant nothing to anybody else, but would mean freedom to Athan Carras.

After a while, Ti-Jean came with a bowl of rice and shredded vegetables, along with another fish and a couple of bananas. Carras was ravenous and ate it all. When he asked for something to drink, he was offered another plastic bottle and, thinking it was water again, took a deep swallow before he discovered that it was a raw and fiery rum, that must have been aged no longer than it took to distill the coarse molasses. It was easily hundred proof. His eyes watered and his nose ran, but Ti-Jean urged him to drink more.

Carras tried to wave the bottle away, but the Haitian shook his gray head. "*Tout,*" he said. All. "*Atò ou dòmi.*" Then you sleep. When Carras pretended not to understand, Ti-Jean pillowed his head on joined hands in the universal mime. "*Dòmi lon tan.*" Sleep a long time.

Carras sighed and signaled assent. Obviously, a strong dose of overproof liquor was part of the plan to keep the prisoner in his makeshift cell. Escape would be harder in an alcoholic stupor. Carras realized that he had to go along with the plan, had to feign timorousness until he had an opportunity. He drained the bottle, and even with the food in his belly he felt the rum taking hold.

Using mime and a basic sound effect, he conveyed to the Haitian that he needed to use a toilet. The man said *"D'acc,"*—Okay—but first he took away the bowl and bottle and locked the door, returning with Falardeau. By now the liquor was clouding Carras's mind, and he had to be helped up the hill to an outhouse beside the cinder block house that must be Falardeau's.

The privy was a far cry from a spotless North American bathroom, but was not as foul as Carras might have feared. There was an actual seat above the hole and even toilet paper—not pillowy soft but better than scratchy newspaper. And there was a bag of lime in the corner to throw into the pit when he was finished. Through the gathering fumes of alcohol, Carras thought about it and the answer came. Falardeau, for all his rough edges, must be solicitous of his pregnant wife's comfort.

They let him wash his hands at a stand pipe next to the house. He looked up and managed to focus eyes that were starting to see things in duplicate and saw Madame Falardeau, her belly swollen almost it seemed to the point of bursting, standing in the doorway of the house, watching them. Before the rum ruined his ability to think, he decided to test his belief in the overseer's concern for his wife. *"Vôtre femme,"* he said, and noticed that the words came out slurred, *"combien de mois?"* How many months pregnant is she?

He watched the way the overseer's eyes went to the woman, thought he saw a tinge of disquiet there. *"Huit,"* the man said.

"Huit?" Carras blinked and held up eight fingers. *"Très grande."* She was very big indeed for eight months.

"Tu es medécin, toi?" said Falardeau.

"Yeah, *oui,"* said Carras, patting his chest with a wet hand. "Me doctor."

Falardeau asked if he had delivered babies. Carras said he had, then added *"Beaucoup bébé,"* mispronouncing it as bookoo beebee. Many babies. It wasn't true lately, but once it had been. He said it again, then laughed at the sound of it, and realized he was very, very drunk.

He struggled to focus on Falardeau. The overseer looked as if he wanted to pursue the discussion further. Obviously he was concerned for his wife, and just as obviously that concern was warring with some other priority. Through the gathering fog in his mind, Carras thought he saw fear there more than avarice. It seemed a not unlikely mix of emotions for someone who was doing Terry Flynnt's bidding.

"Bookoo," he said again, and laughed. Then he found that his legs had become distant and unreliable. Slowly, like a circus bear performing a trick, he sat down on the ground then leaned dangerously backward.

"Night, night," he said. Ti-Jean caught his head before it hit the ground, but Carras didn't know it.

Chapter 11

Carras woke before dawn. They had taken back the clothes he had been given, stripped him naked again. His head was still thick with the rum and he shivered in the clueless darkness of the shed while he strove to remember where he was and what had happened. Then it came back and he sat up, felt around the hard-packed floor for the water bottle.

His hand closed around the neck of a plastic jug but when he lifted it he found it was empty. He groaned. He needed water, needed to rehydrate his tissues or he'd be in even worse trouble when the sun came up. He dropped the empty container and searched through the blackness and found a full bottle. He drank and kept drinking, even though his belly threatened to send the liquid right back up.

Now he sat back against the wall. He ached. His lower back and thighs hurt worst, then the shoulders and arms. His hands, though saved from blistering by the gloves, were sore; they wanted to half close like claws and stretching them open made the tendons complain. His bladder was uncomfortably full but he fought the urge to fill the empty jug. Better to let the water he had just drunk permeate his alcohol-dried system. He didn't want to start a full day of stoop labor with a raging hangover headache.

He rolled over on his hands and knees and crawled to where he expected the door to be. He was off by more than a foot. He felt the rough planks and knew that they were too thick for him to break. Besides, even if he could smash through with kicks from his bare feet the noise would bring Falardeau and the men.

He'd need a quiet way of getting out. He slipped his fingers into the space between the door and the jamb and found that the former was loose in its frame. There was a bar of flat iron across the door. One end of the bar was pierced by a bolt sunk into one of the shed's corner posts. The free end of the bar fitted into a metal hasp on the other corner post. The bar went up and down like the gate on a railroad crossing. A heavy chain secured its free end to the hasp.

The locking mechanism was primitive but effective. The chain meant he couldn't tear his plastic jug apart, slide a piece of it through the crack of the door and lift the bar free. But he thought there was a way to get out. All he needed was a pointed piece of metal and enough time.

When the pressure in his bladder was too much to bear, Carras filled the empty jug and put it in a far corner of the shed. Then he made himself as comfortable on the burlap as its roughness and his pains would let him and went back to sleep.

The second day was harder. They started early and he was stiff and sore from the first day's work. His hangover was not as bad as it might have been but he made a point of holding his head and dry retching when the little boy brought him a bowl filled with some kind of hot porridge. Feigning lack of appetite, he nonetheless cleaned the bowl and licked the spoon. He wanted all the energy he could get, in case the chance to run came along.

It didn't. Falardeau and Ti-Jean watched him closely and the other men also stayed nearby, each keeping an eye trained in Carras's direction. He doubted that any one of them was working to a cane cutter's normal speed. Their main job was to surround and guard the prisoner.

So he stooped and pulled and cut, then stooped and pulled and cut again, always with his eye on the ground in case somebody might have once dropped a nail or a spoon or any small metal implement that a shanghaied doctor might tuck into an armpit and take home to his humble shack. But he might as well have been watching for a surgical scalpel; the ground held nothing but stones and cane roots and the droplets of Carras's sweat that fell like a highly localized rain to the dry soil.

His hands still hurt and his back still ached, but as the morning wore on his muscles warmed to the exercise and his discomfort became tolerable. He let his captors believe otherwise, however, moaning from time to time and frequently stopping to sip water from a bottle they'd given him. By lunch time he was feeling not too bad, but let them think he had to force down the pottage of vegetables, rice and beans they all shared. Like the others, he stretched out in the shade of the banana trees and pulled his leaf hat down over his eyes, but instead of sleeping he watched.

Falardeau was worried, Carras saw, but not about his prisoner. A few times during the morning, he had noticed the overseer looking back up the hill toward the houses. After eating the man did not sleep but sat on the flatbed of the truck, drumming his fingers on the boards beside him. Every few moments he would turn his head and look up the slope and now Carras saw him stiffen.

"*Mesye! Mesye!*" The voice was high pitched and growing louder as the little boy raced down the rutted track. Falardeau jumped down from the flatbed and grabbed the hurtling child.

"*Étan?*" the overseer asked. Is it time?

They boy nodded.

Falardeau wasted no time. "Ti-Jean" he called. "*Gade li!*" Watch him.

The black man was already on his feet. The child had woken everybody. "*Ben sur,*" he said, turning his eyes to Carras.

The doctor sat up, looking suitably confused and saw Falardeau leap into the camion's cab and drive away down the track. They all watched him go, then Ti-Jean said, "*Travay.*" Work.

Barely five minutes passed before the truck came back, Falardeau grinding the gears as he put it at the slope. Carras stood and stretched as it went by and saw a gray haired black woman in the passenger seat beyond the overseer.

"*Travail!*" came Ti-Jean's voice and Carras stooped and seized another armful of sugar cane.

The sun hadn't even touched the hills that formed the western horizon when Ti-Jean called a halt. Falardeau had not come back with the truck so they stacked the cut cane and left it lying. Carras turned over his knife and gloves once more then they walked upslope, the prisoner in the middle of the group.

Falardeau was not to be seen. Ti-Jean gestured Carras toward the shed with the bar on its door. As he had the night before, Carras mimed a need for a toilet and the black man assented and escorted him to the privy.

Sober this time, Carras sat on the toilet seat and ran his eyes carefully over the inside of the outhouse. But he saw nothing that could be adapted to his desire to escape. He thought briefly about hurling a handful of the powdered lime into Ti-Jean's face and making a break for it, but he was sure the others would swiftly run him down. Besides, he had no wish to hurt anyone if he could avoid it; they were not his enemies, just tools in more powerful hands.

He went out to the pump to wash his hands. From here he was close enough to the open door of Falardeau's house to hear the sounds that were coming from within. As Carras had expected, he heard the unmistakable noises of a woman in heavy labor: a high pitched wail almost like an alley cat working its way up to a fight, then heavy sobbing breaths, a gulp of air and again the woman's voice climbing into a keening moan.

The contractions were close. By the way Falardeau had acted since the morning, Carras suspected that the man's wife had been in labor all day. She had looked to be a strong young woman; if she hadn't had the child by now, something was probably wrong.

Ti-Jean took him back to the hut and locked him in. A few minutes later one of the other women brought him a bowl of the vegetable stew and another bottle of water. Carras ate and drank, pausing to listen. Even from here he could hear the sounds from the cinder block house, and he was not hearing the cry of a newborn.

Ti-Jean came after a while and took Carras's bowl and spoon, but there was no bottle of rum to be forced down. Carras sat on his sacking, his back against the rough planks, listening and waiting. The sun went down and the shed grew dark and the sounds from the house became weaker.

It was full night when the clinking of the chain links woke Carras from a doze. Yellow light shone around the edges of the door then flooded the rectangle of the frame as Ti-Jean yanked it open.

"*Viens!*" he said. Come. Carras got to his feet.

The light in Falardeau's house came from a kerosene pressure lantern hung from the living room ceiling which lit the room as brightly as a two hundred watt bulb. His wife was in a small bedroom visible through an open door. She was sitting on a low stool, two women behind her to support her weight, the gray haired black woman squatting between her open thighs. The pregnant woman's head was tilted back against the belly of one of the women. Her eyes were closed and rivulets of sweat ran down her corded throat to soak the simple shift that was her only garment.

Falardeau himself was in the doorway of the little room as Ti-Jean brought Carras in. The overseer's face was like that of a little boy afraid of a spanking. "*M'sieur le docteur,*" he said. "*Pour l'amour de Dieu.*" For the love of God.

The man had imprisoned him, pointed a gun at him, threatened him with a whipping and forced him to work like a field slave. But Carras had an older adversary in this small house, a familiar enemy that was stretching its shadowy hand over the exhausted woman and the life struggling to free itself from her womb. He looked about him. There was a good sized table in the kitchen. He spoke to the women. "*Sur la table, vite!*"

He swept the table clean of plates and cups, sending them crashing to the floor. With Falardeau's help, the neighbors placed the pregnant woman on the table. Carras spoke to them—"*Savon! De l'eau!*"—and they brought him soap and a bowl of water.

While he washed and rinsed his hands he ran his eyes over the patient.

She was unconscious, obviously exhausted. He lifted the hem of the shift and exposed her swollen abdomen, then bent her knees into a position approximating the stirruped delivery posture common in American maternity hospitals.

It had been a long time since Carras had delivered a baby. In fact, the last one he had brought into the world was at the Schweitzer Hospital here in Haiti, more than twenty years ago. But there was no time to contemplate irony. This birth was not going well.

He put his ear to the lower slope of the distended abdomen's dome and listened. Even without a stethoscope he could faintly hear a fetal heartbeat. The child inside was alive, but it wasn't in good shape. The pulse should have been rapid—180 beats a minute—but Carras's estimate was no more than 145. The baby was in distress.

He inserted two fingers inside the woman's vagina. The cervix was fully effaced; she was dilated enough to deliver. But his probing fingers told him the story. Instead of the smooth crown of an infant's head, he felt a tiny foot. The baby was breach.

He gently pushed the foot back the way it had come. It might be possible to turn the fetus in the womb and bring the head into proper alignment with the girdle of pelvic bones that surrounded the mouth of the uterus. But the foot would not go that way. Even as he pressed, another contraction squeezed the woman's womb and the baby's foot extended farther into her birth canal.

He looked at the gray-haired midwife. "*Je dois la couper,*" he said. "*J'ai besoin d'un couteau.*" I must cut her. I need a knife.

The old woman placed a cloth bundle on the table and spread its folds to reveal the contents. There was a small bone handled knife with a blade of stained carbon steel and—Thank God, Carras thought—what looked to be an actual curved needle and suturing thread. She must have acquired them from some clinic. There was even a small bottle of sterilizing alcohol.

She would use the knife to cut umbilical cords and perhaps to perform an amateur episiotomy if necessary to prevent a delivering mother's flesh from tearing. He picked it up and tested the blade's edge on his thumb. It was no scalpel but it was sharp enough to do the job.

But with a silent *Forgive me* to the exhausted patient, Carras showed the little knife to Falardeau and said, "*Y a quelque chose meilleur?*" Got anything better?

The overseer rushed to a cupboard and came back with a plastic container of cutlery, including several knives of different sizes. Carras picked up one after another, examined each closely then set them down on the table. Then, with a noise of impatience, he took up the midwife's tool, poured alcohol on both sides of the blade and rubbed more of it into his fingers.

"*Toi aussi,*" he said to the midwife, indicating the soap and water. She began to wash her hands. To the other women, he said, "*Tenez-la,*" and saw them gather about Falardeau's unconscious wife and put their hands on her arms and shoulders. Their eyes were round and their cheeks drawn. "*Elle sera bien,*" he told them, She'll be all right. He hoped it was true.

Carras pulled the pregnant woman's shift up to her breasts and cleaned the lower slope of her abdomen with the alcohol. Normally, the incision for a caesarian section is made below the "bikini line" of the patient's pubic hair—which is shaved off for the operation—so that when the thatch grows back the scar is not visible. But there was no time for niceties now. Carras put the tip of the little knife to the ligne negre, the dark line of pigmented skin that runs down the abdomen of every pregnant woman, and made a long vertical incision.

The stretched skin and muscle peeled back and the unconscious woman moved on the table. Carras said, "*Tenez-la!*" again to the women and saw them press down hard. He heard Falardeau gasp and swear, but now Carras had no thought for anything but the lives he meant to save. He cut through the midline fascia, the bluish-white connective tissue that sheathes muscle, and there beneath the peritoneum was the purplish red of the overripe uterus.

Blood was seeping into the open wound. From the old woman's kit he took a pad of cloth that looked to be clean and dabbed at the skin bleeders—the veins and arteries severed by his incision. Then he handed the pad to the midwife and said, "*Toi, fais la même.*" You do the same.

Now he dragged the knife through the wall of the womb itself, careful not to cut the contents. The bleeding became heavier and he signaled the old woman to keep dabbing.

Falardeau's wife moaned and one of her feet moved. If she came to while the procedure was unfinished they would have to hold her down. Carras put his hand into the rent of her womb and moved it about until he recognized the shape of a baby's back. He cupped the child's rump so that the head lay upon his forearm and slid the infant out.

He turned the child upside down to clear its airway then slapped it gently on the buttocks. A faint cry was heard. Carras turned the child over and swept his eyes over it. All normal. He looked for Falardeau and said, "*Un p'tit garçon. Ton fils.*" A little boy. Your son.

The overseer was back against the wall of the kitchen. Now his eyes filled with tears. Carras placed the baby on his mother's chest and bent to the task of closing her up.

But as he proceeded to bathe the needle and thread in alcohol he saw a movement in the incision. He set down the suturing equipment and put his hand back into the womb and brought out another son for the Falardeaus. Again he got the child breathing and laid it upon the mother's chest. He saw Falardeau's mouth fall open. The overseer said a word that was half swallowed by emotion, then buried his streaming face in his hands.

I should have expected twins from the breach presentation and the size of the belly, Carras thought, but consoled himself with the recognition that he had had other things on his mind. He showed the midwife how to use her fingers and thumbs to apply pressure on the uterine wall and quickly sutured the incision closed, from bottom to top, using a baseball stitch. *Easier than hearts,* he told himself.

The mother was a good coagulator and the bleeding was quickly stemmed once the uterus was whole again. A minute later and the fascia was reconnected, a minute after that the skin was closed. "*Tout fait,*" Carras said. All done.

The mother was waking. A deeper color was showing itself beneath her cafe-au-lait-colored skin. No sign of shock, Carras noted. Rest and fluids and a third world immune system would see her through. She was beginning to stir, no doubt in response to the two infants that cried and moved on her breast. Carras caught the eye of the midwife and moved his hand in a way that said, *All yours.*

She smiled, revealing that she had no more than four teeth.

"*M'sieur le docteur,*" Falardeau said.

Dr. Athan Carras, deliverer of babies under trying circumstance, was so in the moment that he opened his mouth to say, "*Ça ne fait rien,*"—Think nothing of it—and was surprised to feel Ti-Jean's rock hard grip close around his upper arm. Falardeau had the grace at least to look embarrassed as he said, "*Je le regrets...*"

But, sorry or not, he was sending Carras back to his shed with the iron bar across the door. The doctor gave the overseer a look that invited the man to feel all the shame he could muster. Then he shrugged and let Ti-Jean lead him back into captivity.

But when the door was shut, the bar in place and the chain snugged to its hook, Carras sat back against the wall and smiled. He took out the paring knife he had slipped into the pocket of his shorts and hid it beneath the sacking. Outside he could hear the celebrations beginning at chez Falardeau.

Ti-Jean and Falardeau came back after a little while. Again the overseer was apologetic but he still made Carras give up his clothes and required him to drink the overproof rum. But his captors were both well along the road to full inebriation and did not notice that Carras managed to spill a good portion of the raw liquor while making a flamboyant toast to the newborns. He managed to waste more of it by insisting that Falardeau and Ti-Jean take a drink from his bottle, a kindness which each accepted with gestures of courteous appreciation.

The bottle was not even drunk down when they escorted Carras back into his shed and lowered the bar to seal him in. He put his ear against the wall and heard the chain rattling against its hooks, then the voices of both men receding toward the cinder block house singing a jaunty kreyol song whose chorus ended in *bom, bom, bom!* followed by a word Carras could not make out.

No sooner were they on their way than Carras thrust two fingers down his throat and vomited up the rum in his stomach. Then he recovered his paring knife and applied it to the wall near the corner post where the hook that held the chain was set. The sides of the horizontal planks met each other without gaps but his sensitive fingers were able to find the edge of one, at about the height of the hook and chain. He cut a sliver as long as his hand from it, then took one from the plank that abutted from above. The wood was not hard and soon he could feel a gap between the two planks wide enough to put his fingers into.

He stopped and listened. There were more voices raised in song at Falardeau's house, men's and women's, and he could hear a drum tapping behind the singers. Carras cut again, though his overworked hands had begun to ache as he gripped the small handle. He took another splinter, then stopped to flex his fingers and pull them until the knuckles cracked.

The party at the overseer's was growing louder. Carras doubted that he would be checked again that night and settled himself to work slowly. He smiled grimly to himself. The renowned cardiothoracic surgeon with the wall full of honorific plaques and testimonial letters was crouched naked in a rough shack in rural Haiti, carving a hole in a wall.

The planks were a little more than an inch thick, but as the gap between them steadily widened Carras avoided piercing them all the way to the outside. He would remove wood from the inner surfaces until he had a space wide enough to put his hand and arm through; only then would he break completely through to the outside. He didn't want anyone to pass by and notice the hole before it was big enough to be useful. He would not get a chance like this again.

As he cut and tore away wood he thought about the next step. The only vehicle was Falardeau's camion, the keys to which might be in the ignition or in the overseer's pocket. Even if he could get the truck started he had no idea how far he might get in it. The gas tank could well be empty; Falardeau didn't look the type to purchase full tanks of expensive gasoline—he seemed more the two-dollar fill-up kind.

Besides, the absence of the truck might be noticed immediately, and Carras's plan was to be far away before he was missed. Everyone would sleep late tomorrow and if he could contrive to leave the shed looking normal perhaps no one would check the prisoner until well after sun up.

He cut another splinter then stopped and flexed his hand. He had now created a wide depression along both sides of the two planks where they joined.

He lightly tapped the wood that remained between him and the outside. It rang hollow. Not far to go now.

He listened. The noise from the house was louder, the voices more raucous. A guitar had joined the drum and there was a rhythmic percussion of bare feet on a wooden floor. They were dancing. But when people danced, especially when the combined exertion with rum, they got hot, and when they got hot they came outside for fresh, night-cooled air.

He did not need someone to be standing on Falardeau's front step, with light from the pressure lantern flooding out to at least partly illuminate the shed, when he broke through the wall, untied the chain and lifted the iron bar. He cut another length of wood from the inside of the lower plank but had to admit that the job was all but done. He began lightly scoring the thin outer layer, so that it would come out quickly and quietly, and thought again about the next step.

They might expect him to go down the track and into the banana groves, since he knew his way that far at least. But his mind came back to the light plane of the day before. If he went over the hill and kept going, he would come to where the plane had landed. There must be at least a farm there, maybe a town, perhaps even a rural police station from which he could make a radiophone call to the US consulate.

He imagined himself walking naked up to a farm house in the middle of the pitch black Haitian night and felt around in the darkness for the sacking that had been his bed. He pulled the heap apart and found that there were half a dozen different sacks.

One was newer than the others, judging by its feel and smell. It was about four feet long and two feet broad, open at one end. Carras cut a hole in the middle of the closed end, wide enough to accept his head, and a hole at each adjacent corner for his arms. He wriggled his way into the rudimentary garment. It itched but it covered the essentials.

He wished they hadn't taken his sandals. But he cut the other sacks into strips and wound these around his feet and ankles, splitting and tying the ends of the lengths of burlap the way the old first aid manuals had taught him to do bandages when he was a Boy Scout.

Guess I'm as prepared as I'm going to be, he thought. He sat with his back against the wall and listened. The noise from Falardeau's party gave no indication that it would soon cease, and he composed himself to wait.

In the darkness, with only the music to catch his awareness, his mind wandered through the events of the past weeks. When he looked back on his life before all this, back to his routine of surgery and teaching, it all seemed now like some brightly lit but tightly confined scene viewed through the wrong end of a telescope.

He had thought that the struggle to develop and perfect the heart-and-a-half procedure had been a challenge. Then into his life had come Terry Flynnt. But now Carras was going to overcome that challenge too. He thought of Flynnt, how hard and unbending he was. He would like to introduce the man to Charlie Vance, and say to his friend, *You think I'm a Puritan, all black or white thinking? Take a look at this guy.*

But as he thought about it he decided he ought to be perversely grateful to Flynnt. Carras had needed a challenge. Not playing one-upmanship games with James Bonar Auldfield or writing applications to foundations for penny ante grants, not even reconnecting with his lost son and ex-wife, though that was still something he had to do. It was true that Hilary Cartiere and the research institution had been a temptation, but it was the kind of temptation that that wily old Greek Odysseus had faced when he'd washed up on the island of don't-worry-be-happy lotus-eaters, the trap of ease and torpor. No, Carras saw, what he'd really needed was what always made him come most alive—a real-life, balls to the wall contest. Flynnt had given him one, and Carras meant to win it. Afterwards, he would sort out the other problems in his life, and everything would be fine.

He laughed softly and, listening to his own sound, realized that the noise from Falardeau's had softened. He got to his knees and used the knife to bore a small hole through the outer layer of the plank. He put an eye to the puncture and peered up at the overseer's house.

The pressure lantern had been put out; there was only the yellowy light of oil lamps. People were leaving, walking down into the darkness in twos or threes, calling to each other and laughing The drum had stopped and he saw a man with a guitar upended over his shoulder, coming down the track and stepping with the exaggerated care of the thoroughly intoxicated.

The guitar player passed the shed, humming something. A few more shapes were silhouetted against the yellow glow from Falardeau's, then there was only stillness. A moment later, the last light was blown out and there was only the scant illumination of the massed stars.

Carras waited a few more minutes then, feeling with his fingers, he carefully slid the point of the knife along the groove he had scored in the remaining veneer of wood that had been the lower plank. A thin lath of wood a little larger than his hand came away from the bottom plank. A few seconds later he had carved away a similar sized piece from the upper plank, creating a hole large enough for his arm to pass through.

The gap was above the iron bar and only a foot from where the restraining chain was wound around the hook. He unwound it and pulled it through the hole. Now he slid the knife through the crack between door and jamb and lifted the bar free. He had to run the blade all the way up the side and across the top of the door before it would open enough to let him slip out.

He lowered the bar back into place, rewound the chain on its hook and replaced the wood, pressing the pieces into the gaps they had come from to leave the wall looking unbroken.

Then, walking quietly on his burlap wrapped feet, Carras stole up the hill, past Falardeau's sleeping house. There was a vegetable garden, with a low wire fence to keep out chickens, and he crossed it carefully. Beyond, the slope rose to the crest of the hill and when he was over that, he began to feel his way down the other side.

The burlap wraps, while protecting him from sharp stones, didn't offer much traction and after a couple of near spills, arms windmilling as he fought for footing and balance, Carras opted for sliding down the slope on his buttocks. The dim starlight let him see vague shapes from the corners of his vision but anything he tried to focus on remained masked in darkness.

He made good time, however, because Haiti's original tropical forest had long since been cut down for commercial use or for fuel to cook the meals of the poor. There was nothing that was worth fencing or walling in on these barren hills and he found that if he tilted his head to one side he could see well enough to maintain a reasonable walking speed.

At the bottom of the first slope he found a narrow valley—not much more than a draw—and within a few minutes he was across it and ascending the next hill. He was tired but he established a good rhythm and kept at it.

Over the next hill the ground evened out into a stretch of very faintly sloping land that seemed to go on and on. He came across no fences, but gradually it dawned on him that he must be in a pasture; he could smell cattle dung. For a moment he worried about stepping in a cow pat, then laughed. It certainly wouldn't spoil his footwear.

He was still chuckling about it when he walked smack into something large, warm and at least chest high. He bounced off, startled, sat down on the ground, then leapt back up immediately as the night exploded in a rush of snorts, bellows and pounding hooves. From the corners of his eyes, he saw dark moving shapes on either side and he yelled and waved his arms, hoping that the animals could see him better than he could see them. It was one thing to walk into a dozing cow, another thing all together to be run down by a panicked herd of beef.

He listened to the stampede's diminishing sounds and resumed walking in what he hoped was his original direction. He realized that he should have been trying to keep a bearing by noting the positions of the constellations, some of which he wasn't sure he recognized this far south. As he went forward, looking at the horizon, he saw some of the lower stars abruptly disappear. He went farther and saw more of the bright pinpoints swallowed by something dark and bulky and irregular in shape.

He turned his head to look from the corner of one eye. Trees, he thought, and where there are trees and cattle there should be a farm. He went forward faster now and before too long he became aware of something that was definitely man-made stretching off to either side of him. When he went forward, hands outstretched before him, he found a chain-link fence, and when he reached up it was taller than he was.

"Yes!" he said, under his breath. A fence of this quality meant that the farm it surrounded was no mere hovel next to a half-acre vegetable patch. This was the home of a relatively rich Haitian; chances were good it would contain some way of communicating with the world—a radio or radiophone. Carras need only find the gate and call out to be admitted.

He followed the fence to his right. It went on a long way and his hopes rose higher. Someone with a farmhouse and outbuildings this extensive might even have a satellite phone.

The fence finally turned a corner. Here the ground outside was no longer pasture. With his peripheral vision, Carras saw a wide dark strip. A road, he thought, but when he went to investigate he found it was not asphalt but hard packed soil running straight in either direction. Not far off there was a gray shape where the dark strip ended.

It was strange that he could see that far, Carras thought. When he turned back toward the fence, looking straight on, he could almost make it out. He looked up at the sky and saw a lightening of the darkness down at the far end of the earthen road where it cut between more trees.

The moon, he thought and even as he formed the words in his mind, the first yellowy sliver of light rose almost at the end of the road. No, not a road—it's an airstrip. When he looked to the crude runway's other end he saw that the gray object was the light plane he had seen the day before.

This was the farm he'd hypothesized. Dr. Athan Carras had come back to civilization.

He decided to wait until the moon was well up then search for a gate in the fence. He watched as the glowing orb rose sedately into the sky, its early gold becoming first silver then white as it climbed. When it was completely clear of the horizon, Carras looked to the fence and noticed that it was topped along its entire length with razor wire.

"That's funny," he said aloud and the sound of his voice prompted a deep *wuff!* from somewhere beyond the fence. The first bark was followed by another, then other dogs took up the alarm. There were many of them, and they sounded big and not friendly.

A light came on somewhere through the trees beyond the fence—a bright light, the kind that nervous homeowners install on their garages and front walks in high crime areas. Another light came on, and now the dogs were going crazy.

He heard a door open then someone was yelling at the animals. The volume of the canine riot dropped, and Carras was about to call out, "*Au secours!*" the French for help, when he realized that the voices he was hearing were not French or Kreyol. They were Spanish.

His Spanish was rusty. He knew *Ayudame, por favor* was the same as *au secours* and he was going to try that when some part of him finally made the connection: Spanish voices; razor wire; vicious dogs; an airstrip and a small plane out in the middle of nowhere.

This was no farm. This was a way station on the cocaine highway from Colombia across the Caribbean to America. The shouting men would not help him contact the authorities. They would shoot him and feed him to the monsters who were baying for his blood.

Carras ran for the only cover he could see—the plane. He raced around its tail which stood as tall as he was and froze there, gasping for breath and listening. He heard more Spanish and the sound of metal ringing against metal, followed by the skitter of clawed paws on hard earth.

They had let the dogs out.

Chapter 12

Carras had once seen a rabbit run down by a dog. The prey had had a fifty-foot lead but the pursuer, one of those big yellow mongrels that make lovable pets, closed the gap in seconds. Though the rabbit jinked and dodged, the dog ran it down, sank its long fangs into the doomed animal's hindquarters and with a blur of head shakes tore the rabbit almost in half. When the teeth sank in, the victim let loose a high-pitched shriek that had pierced Carras's heart. He'd had no idea rabbits could scream.

In peak condition and wearing two-hundred-dollar Nikes, Carras knew he could not have outrun a pack of dogs. Exhausted and with rags on his feet, the best he could hope for was that the men would shoot him before the animals could do much damage.

He heard a *skriek* of unoiled hinges as the gate opened. The dogs had stopped barking. They were making an eager gobbling sound, their claws clicking and scrabbling on the hard pack. Their noses had told them where he was. They were coming.

Carras moved out of the cover of the small plane's tail and tried the handle on the door. It opened. He found the little corrugated steel footstep and climbed in, closing the door behind him. A second later a big, dark domed skull appeared at the side window and Carras instinctively flinched as the Rottweiler growled. He heard its claws futilely scratching for purchase on the plane's metal skin then the dog's head slid sideways and disappeared. Almost immediately it was back.

Carras peered through the window toward the house. The men had not come out of the gate but they would eventually. Right now there was time to think. The moonlight was growing stronger and Carras could see the plane's controls and instrument panel. It was some kind of Cessna, similar but not identical to the one he had flown in several times with Charlie Vance.

There was a short burst of gunfire from the house, the burr of an automatic weapon and a tongue of flame pointing upward through the darkness. Somebody yelled in Spanish and there was a second burst, then silence.

Carras had seen Vance start his plane enough times. He felt along the instrument panel where the ignition key ought to be, and there it was. But he knew Vance's plane didn't start by a turn of the key; there was something else that had to be done first.

He remembered. Down on the left was a flat black switch that turned on the plane's electrical system. He put his left hand on the switch and gripped the key with his right. Then he paused. If he turned on the electrics, any lights that had been left on would immediately come up. The men at the house would have no doubt where the intruder was.

Carras took a deep breath, let it out and worked the switch and key in rapid succession. The panel lit up and the navigation lights on wing and tail came on, and the propeller began to turn—but only haltingly.

Over its stuttering he heard the dogs barking furiously and another yell from the house. There was a second blast of gunfire, this time the shots whirring over the plane. He was praying that they would shoot up their own aircraft only as a last resort.

Focus! Carras told himself. *What does Charlie do?*

Now he remembered: the fuel mixture control. It was like a manual choke on the old time cars his dad had fixed in the service station on Market Street. He groped and found the rod with the knob on it and pulled it toward him. Immediately the engine's voice deepened and the propeller spun faster.

Now the throttle, he said. It should be down and to the right of the yoke. He reached and it was there. He pulled it all the way out and the plane began to roll forward. He thanked God the drug runners had been too lazy to put chocks under the wheels.

He could also be thankful that the plane was already pointed down the runway because he wasn't sure how to steer. Again he tried for a mental picture of what his friend did, saw it in his mind's eye. It was pedals on the floor—right foot, left foot—that moved the rudder on the tail. He felt for them with his rag-swathed feet, tried a little pressure on one then the other, felt the accelerating plane lazily veer to one side then the other. *I can steer!*

The plane was steadily tending toward the left side of the dirt track. *They do that,* he remembered Vance saying—*the propellers' rotation pulls the plane to one side.* He eased his foot down on the right rudder pedal and the Cessna straightened out.

He was picking up speed. He was already passing the gate and now more lights came on, somebody training a spotlight on the plane. He turned his eyes away, to keep from being blinded, but still saw the flame of the automatic weapon at the corner of his vision.

The gunman was not shooting high this time. Carras heard bullets striking the fuselage behind him and felt a momentary chill of terror in case a fuel tank was hit.

There was another burst of fire and he saw a spark beside him as a round ricocheted off a wing spar. Then the Cessna was hurtling forward, bouncing on its wheels as if it had a will of its own and couldn't wait to get into the air. Carras recognized the sensation from flying with Vance; it was time to pull back on the yoke. He grabbed the two vertical handles and drew them slowly toward him as he had seen his friend do. The bouncing stopped. He was climbing.

He held the yoke back, feeling the plane's ascent grow steeper. His stomach sank toward his backbone and he saw the air opening up around him as the land fell away. *Up and away,* he thought. *Charlie's right, this is great.*

He felt a brief tremor in the airframe. Then came another shudder, this one stronger, shaking the yoke in his hands. The plane lurched in the air like a car whose engine was about to stall. Had the gunfire damaged the machine? Was the motor about to quit and drop him to the ground?

No, the engine was roaring at its top rpms. But now the tremor was becoming a shudder. And there was something wrong with the lift. He could feel it in his belly, like he was coming to the first rise at the top of a roller coaster, that stillness before the fall into the down slope.

High school physics saved him. He could see it in his memory: the diagram showing an airfoil in cross section. The air flowing over the wing went faster than the air going underneath: that provided lift. But angle the airfoil too sharply and all the lift went away. If the airfoil was the wing of an airplane the plane stopped flying. It stalled and fell out of the air.

Carras eased the yoke forward and the shuddering stopped. The plane continued to lift smoothly toward the moon that had risen above the end of the runway. He let it climb until he thought he must be over a mile high then pushed the yoke forward some more until he leveled off.

Flying toward the rising moon meant that he was heading roughly east. A small compass set on top of the instrument panel confirmed his course. He thought about that: east would take him to the Dominican Republic, which shared the island of Hispaniola with Haiti. That was too close for Carras to feel comfortable. The Haitian military had been steady customers for Terry Flynnt—Carras was sure that Falardeau the banana grower and part-time slave driver was ex-military—and Carras would bet that Flynnt had plenty of old friends among the Dominicans, who were only marginally less corrupt than the Haitians.

He struggled to remember his Caribbean geography. To the north was Florida but it would be at the extreme range of this plane. He peered at the instruments, searching for the fuel gauge. There were two of them, one registering full and the other three-quarters. He didn't know how far that would take him, and now that he was thinking of it he eased in the throttle an inch or so—Vance always did that once he was at cruising altitude. It would save gas and increase his flight range.

Northwest was Cuba where he might be shot down by a nervous military. To the northeast and maybe to the north was a spray of little islands that gradually worked their way up to the Bahamas—the name came to him now: the Turks and Caicos. They were British protectorates, which meant they were governed by laws, not men in sunglasses and sweaty uniforms who would clap an errant doctor in jail for a modest bribe and hold him until Flynnt's men showed up to take him somewhere even worse than Falardeau's.

Carras turned the yoke left and the plane banked. When the compass said he was heading northeast he leveled the controls again. But the plane kept turning. A cold sweat broke out on his torso under the itching burlap. Again he was frightened that the gunfire might have damaged the controls. Gently, he turned the yoke to the right and let go the breath he had been holding. The plane straightened and flew level.

By careful experimentation, he worked out how to turn and level off again. But the maneuvers had caused him to lose altitude. He was out over the sea now, the coast of Hispaniola a dark blur behind him, the moonlight lying on the water like a glittering cloak. He remembered that Charlie Vance had once said that flying over water at night was the most dangerous. You might think you had hundreds of feet of air beneath you, when all you really had were dozens. Any loss of lift—an air pocket or downdraft—could send him tumbling wing-over-tail to break up in the sea. Chances were he'd be battered into unconsciousness and drowned when the plane sank.

Carras gave the engine more throttle and pulled the yoke back to put the Cessna in a climb. The plane ought to fly with greater fuel efficiency in the thinner air up above, and the higher he was the easier it would be to spot land. He didn't want to think about another factor: if he ran out of gas the higher he was the longer the glide before he came down.

He leveled off at what he thought must be ten thousand feet, and eased in the throttle. The Cessna cut smoothly through tranquil air. Carras looked around for an altimeter. When he found it, it said he was at twelve thousand. The higher the better, he thought again, although his limbs were bare and it was cold in the plane. The thin sacking provided little warmth. He looked for a heater, but if there was one it wasn't obvious. Or maybe it just wasn't working; the plane had a well used look that suggested it was far from new.

He found he didn't need to keep his hands on the yoke, so he rubbed his arms and bare thighs for a while to stimulate circulation then tucked his hands into his armpits. He shivered and looked out at the moon which had now climbed well above the horizon. He and it were the only objects in sight above the sea.

Off to his left there was a faint glow on the horizon that he thought might be Cuba. Ahead he saw nothing but stars and the moonlit flicker of the propeller. To look for an island down on the sea far below he would have to put the plane into a slight dive. He did so now but there was nothing but water all the way to the horizon. He brought the plane back up to twelve thousand feet and leveled off again.

He yawned, a great face splitter followed by another just as big. There was nothing to do but try to keep warm and stay awake. He thought about what he would have to do when it came time to land, trying to conjure up images of what Charlie Vance did when he brought them down. But Carras had always had a queasy feeling about landings; he tended to close his eyes for the last few seconds, not opening them until he felt the comforting bump of wheels on runway.

You were supposed to come in slow but not too slow, he knew. Or you would stall and crash. And you had to angle the nose up at the right time. But not too much or, again, you would stall and crash. Now that he thought about it, he didn't know where the brakes were. If he got down he might not be able to stop the plane.

He shivered and rubbed his thighs again. If he brought the plane to the ground in one piece he'd cut the engine and hope for the best.

He wondered if he should call a mayday, like they did in the movies. Perhaps someone could talk him down. He looked for an earphone and mike headset such as Vance used, but there was nothing like it in the cockpit. He didn't see a hand mike either and realized after poking around that the plane had no radio. The owners didn't trust their mules to talk to anybody once they were in the air.

There was no clock either. He thought it might be as late as five now and wondered what time the sun would come up at this latitude. There didn't seem to be anything but moon to the east although the moonlight could be masking the dawn.

He knew that the thoughts about landing and sunrise were just his way of keeping himself mentally busy. The truth was, he was out over the sea in a plane he didn't know how to bring down. The fuel was being steadily eaten away by the thrumming engine and Carras's memories of flights with Vance left him only a hazy guess as to what the Cessna's range might be—probably no more than five hundred miles on one and three quarters tanks—and he had an even fuzzier grasp as to the location of the nearest land.

These might be his last hours of life, and he was using them to keep busy. Keeping busy was how he always managed to keep from thinking unpleasant thoughts, he admitted to himself. But then he also had to admit that it was a philosophy that hadn't let him down so far. His mind wandered toward Beth and Costas, but he told himself now was not the time to dwell on that situation. He needed positive thoughts, thoughts that would keep him strong.

He reminded himself that yesterday he'd been a slave under the threat of fist and whip. By his own efforts he had freed himself from captivity and now he was twelve thousand feet up above the rest of the world. Maybe he would come down okay, or maybe he would plunge unwitnessed into the unforgiving sea like the boy in the old legend, Icarus, who had cockily flown too close to the sun and melted the wax that held the feathers on his wings.

Carras didn't feel cocky, but despite the cold and his fear that he might not make it through this ordeal, he knew that he had taken all that Terry Flynnt had thrown at him and he had come out the other side with his pride intact.

• • •

Leonard Maigrot was having the bridge dream again. He was running across one of those suspension bridges that were strung across bottomless gorges in adventure movies set in godforsaken places. He could see empty air through the small wooden planks tied to twisted ropes underfoot. The detail in the dream was always sharp: he could see the knots in the wood and the fibers in the skeins of rope. And ahead, where the cable attached to posts dug into the cliff top, he could see the individual strands snapping. If he did not get there soon, the ropes would part and he would fall, twisting and screaming, like the people he had seen from his office after the planes hit the towers.

His bedside phone pulled him out of the dream. He grabbed for the receiver. "What?"

It was Isaac Dumoulin. "Are you awake?"

"Yeah. No, wait." There was sweat on Maigrot's face when he rubbed his eyes. He wiped it away with the sheet and came back to the phone. "Okay," he said.

"Our friend from the plantation called on the satellite phone," Isaac said. "The package is gone."

Maigrot was fully awake now. "Gone? What kind of gone? Your guy didn't... do anything stupid, did he? I told you I didn't like that plantation.

Too many people. Too many eyes and mouths."

"No, the man ran. He got out and took off, I don't know how."

"Well, what are we doing about it?"

"We're looking for him, what do you think?"

"I think the whole fucking thing is coming apart!"

"Calm down," Isaac said. "We'll handle it."

"Where's the boss?"

"On the boat."

Maigrot was getting up. "I'm going to the office," he said. "Meet me there."

At eight thirty-four, Falardeau called again. Maigrot and Isaac took the call on the secure line in the executive vice president's office. Neither of them spoke French, but Falardeau's English coming out of the speaker phone was reasonable.

"I send people to look, we find his foot markings. He got no shoes but cloth on his foot so they look like nobody else. He go over the hill. We follow. We come to a place everybody know about, drug people, *Colombiens*, you understan'?"

"Yeah, go on," Maigrot said.

"We don't go there. Too many gun. But *les indigens*—the people live around there..."

"The neighbors," Maigrot said.

"Yeah, the neighbors they say plenty shooting last night."

"The dopers shot him?"

"Non. They say the dopers plenty mad. Somebody steal their plane."

"Wait a minute," Maigrot said and pushed the hold button. To Isaac, he said, "I didn't see anything in the backgrounder about him flying planes."

"I don't think he knows how."

"He knew enough to get one into the air."

Isaac shrugged. "Doesn't mean he knows how to land it."

"This guy has already given us too many surprises," Maigrot said. "You want to see if he's got another one in his little doctor's bag?"

Isaac nodded. "We can arrange some coverage, just in case he comes down alive. Let's see what Falardeau knows about these Colombians."

• • •

The morning sun poured some warmth into the Cessna's cockpit and that was good, but the glare of light on the eastern sea made it impossible to tell if there was land down there. Carras squinted his eyes against the glitter below but could see nothing.

When he closed his eyes red and gold blobs danced against black. He had to force the lids open again. He'd counted himself exhausted when he'd been trudging across the pasture before moon rise. What he felt now was a fatigue that didn't have a name, but it came with a memory: all those emergency-room shifts when he was a young doctor, sometimes working thirty-six hours with no more than a few twenty-minute naps and endless cups of coffee.

He wouldn't mind some coffee now. He'd searched the cockpit as best he could but it contained nothing to eat or drink. He wished he'd brought the plastic bottle of water from the shed, but he'd been in so much of a hurry to get away that he had left it and the little knife behind.

He swallowed dryly and looked again at the fuel indicators. The right-hand one had read empty for a long time. Now the needle on the left gauge was tapping against empty. He didn't know if that meant he still had a gallon or two or was flying on fumes.

He banked the plane a little to the left then after a moment to the right so that he could look down through the side window. The view was better than through the front and the glittering propeller. Again all he saw was sun dazzle on blue ocean.

Far off to the left was a ship, a freighter it looked like. Carras wondered if perhaps he should head for it, try to put the plane down on the water and get out before it sank. Certainly, the crew would see him and lower a boat.

But he had once watched a TV news clip, from off the coast of Africa somewhere, where a crippled airliner had tried to come down in shallow water. Even in the hands of an expert pilot the aircraft had touched a wingtip to the sea and immediately it had spun and begun to come apart.

If Carras came down hard, pinwheeling across the waves—and the tiny ripples down there must be substantial troughs and crests—he could be battered unconscious in the crash. When the boat arrived from the freighter, they would find nothing but an oil slick.

He waved goodbye to the ship. What he needed was a nice little island with a nice little coastal road, flat and straight. Then he'd line it up and put it down, and if he was still breathing after that there'd be a car to take him to the nearest hospital.

He banked left and right again, squinting against the glare and suddenly there was a darker patch amid the brightness. He rubbed his eyes and looked again and said, slowly but with feeling, "Yabba, dabba, doo."

It was an island, all right. He turned the plane toward the sun and after a few minutes the shape in the water was free of the glare: not too big, only a couple of miles long and maybe half that in width, dark green edged with white, forest and beach and a coral reef out from the shore. If it was a coral island, it would be as flat as it looked.

He was approaching it at almost a ninety degree angle to its length. To land on it, he would have to curve around the nearer end and come in parallel to the shore. He pushed the yoke forward and as the plane began to descend he worked the rudder to angle off to the right. When he thought he had gone far enough he reversed the controls and saw the island ahead and to the left. A little more curve, a little lower descent, and he would be on track.

"I should cut the throttle a bit," he said aloud. His voice sounded parched and crackly around the edges. Just a dry mouth, he thought.

He was lined up now, the plane dropping gradually toward the strip of beach and a gravel road that backed it. *Too steep?* he wondered and pulled on the yoke to flatten the angle of descent, but now he couldn't see very well out the front. He eased the throttle in a little more and pushed the yoke forward.

I can do this, he thought.

The plane's engine sputtered and stopped.

"Uh oh."

He looked out the side window. He was a good hundred and fifty feet in the air. He could see the waves rushing up the shallow beach and a wooden boat out in the water, with a net over the side, two men holding it, standing frozen, watching him. He felt an absurd impulse to wave.

The plane was coming down fast, too fast. The propeller was still turning. Weren't you supposed to feather it? Whatever that meant. Too late for it anyway. Now the beach was coming up, way too fast. The gravel road was stretched out in front of him; he was pretty well lined up.

He pulled back on the yoke. It didn't want to come. He had to brace his feet against the rudder pedals and draw the control toward him. His right hand ached from two days of the cane knife and his arms were trembling with fatigue. He saw the muscles in his forearms jumping of their own accord.

That's it, he told himself. *It either happens or it doesn't.* He thought of Beth and Costas and Charlie Vance. "Wish I'd watched you, Charlie," he said and then it came.

• • •

The two men in the boat saw the plane silently falling toward the empty road. The white man looked at them through the window then the tail of the plane smacked into the road and crumpled. The front wheels hit almost immediately after but they didn't roll.

"Dey jus' broke, mon," Cecil Bingham, owner and captain of the fish boat, told the police sergeant that afternoon. "Den de wing come down and hit de sand, and de whole t'ing..." he rolled one hand over the other like a TV news director telling a newscaster to speed it up. "We t'ink it got to go boom. Mon, in de movies dey all burst into flame. But it stop, upside down on de beach, so we go see how de mon is doing."

"You take anyt'ing out of de plane?" the sergeant said. "You know I goin' to find out if you lie to me, Cecil."

"Ain't nothin' to take," the fisherman said. "Just de white mon in de gunny sack." He scratched his head. "Why de mon dressed like Fred Flintstone?"

• • •

"Dr. Athan Carras," Carras said, not for the first time. "I am Chief of Cardiothoracic Surgery at Yale University. I have no identification because I was kidnaped and had to steal a plane to escape." He had already said the same thing to three black policemen, two of them in white tunics with blue pants, the third in a jaunty straw hat and tropical shirt.

Now he was telling it again to the slim blond man in the well tailored suit who was seated on the folding chair next to Carras's hospital bed. Carras hadn't seen a bed like it in over twenty years. All he wanted to do was sleep in it, but the blond man wouldn't let him.

"And would you tell us from whom you stole the airplane?" the man asked in an accent that sounded to Carras like impeccable Queen's English.

"We were not formally introduced," Carras said. His forehead hurt where he must have hit the edge of the instrument panel, though he didn't remember taking the injury. "It was dark and they were behind barbed wire, a pack of ravening dogs and a machine gun that they were firing in my direction. If I had to guess, I would say they might have been drug smugglers."

"Hmmm," said the Englishman.

"Now would you mind returning the favor?" Carras said.

"I beg your pardon?"

"Would you mind telling me who you are? And where the hell I am?"

"You're in the secure ward of the general hospital on the island of Grand Caicos in the Turks and Caicos Islands. And I am Chief Inspector Matthew Keeling of New Scotland Yard."

"New Scotland Yard?"

There was nothing wrong with the crease in the policeman's pants but he ran a thumb and forefinger along it anyway. "I'm seconded to an anti-drugs task force established in conjunction with your country's Drug Enforcement Agency," he said.

"Well, if you want me to tell you more about the drug smugglers, I don't have much to give you. It was dark and I was escaping from the people who were holding me on the plantation in Haiti."

"Hmmm," said the policeman.

Carras sat up in the hospital bed. It hurt to do it, but he was still surprised that he was able to. He was very lucky not to have woken up wrapped in plaster and strung up from a traction harness. Instead, when he had come to he was strapped to a stretcher in the helicopter that had flown him to this place. He had passed straight through casualty, as the British called their emergency ward, to be brought to this private room with wire netting on the windows. So far he had seen more policemen than medical staff.

"I'd like to see a doctor," he said. "I'd like to know what the diagnosis is."

The Englishman went to the end of the bed and found a chart. He looked it over and said, "Scrapes and contusions, possible concussion. Does that sound right to you, doctor?"

Carras held out his hand and the policeman gave a genteel shrug and passed the chart to him. Carras scanned the notations. He wasn't feeling any of the symptoms that indicated concussion, but there was a bump on his forehead and he had definitely been unconscious. "Yes, it sounds right," he said.

"Hmmm."

The man's tone indicated suspicion. "Do you doubt that I am a doctor?" Carras said.

"Oh, not at all," said Keeling. "You are Dr. Athan Carras of Yale University."

Carras was too tired to raise his voice, but he let his growing anger show. "Then why all the 'Hmmms' and why do I have the feeling that if I try to leave this room you're going to stop me?" Carras said. "Am I under arrest?"

The Englishman twitched his lips then said, "Not as such."

"What the hell does that mean?"

"It means that there are unusual circumstances surrounding your presence in the Turks and Caicos Islands," the policeman said.

"Tell me about it," Carras said.

"I'm sorry?"

"An American expression. It means I already know what you mean."

Keeling seemed glad to have the information. "We found what appears to have been traces of cocaine in the aeroplane," he said.

"I told you, they were probably drug smugglers."

"Hmmm."

"I'm getting fed up with this," Carras said. "A lot of people lately have been making my life difficult, and when I say 'difficult' I am using the kind of understatement that you Brits are supposed to specialize in. I'm not telling you anything more until I see someone from the nearest US consulate."

"Actually," Keeling said. "Someone from your government is on his way to talk to you as we speak."

"Good," said Carras. "Maybe I'll get some answers."

Keeling resumed his seat and folded his hands. He leaned forward with an earnest expression and said, "If I were you, I should expect more questions."

"Such as what? said Carras.

"Such as why your Drug Enforcement Agency is convinced that you are heavily involved in the cocaine traffic."

Chapter 13

I n the image on the computer monitor's screen, the hooded eyes of Frank Mendoza looked straight ahead then flicked toward the camera that must be mounted to the side of his own work station. "That's Athan Carras, all right," he said.

"You're sure," said the balding DEA man in the tropical weight suit, his tone indicating that he didn't want Mendoza to be sure at all.

"I'm sure," Mendoza said.

"And he's head of," the half-bare cranium bent as the man carefully read the words from a piece of paper on the desk in front of him, "cardiothoracic surgery at Yale?"

"Yes, he is. And he was in my office not more than four days ago telling me he might be kidnaped." Mendoza's eyes moved. He would be looking at Carras's video image on his own computer screen in his office at the J. Edgar Hoover Building, a thousand miles away in Washington, DC. "Looks like you were right, doctor."

For the first time since he'd been taken from the hospital room by the two DEA agents, the balding young one and the middle-aged Hispanic one— they hadn't told him their names—Carras felt the tension go out of his overworked back muscles. He looked into the mini-camera on top of the monitor in front of him and said, "I wish I hadn't been, but thank you, Special Agent Mendoza."

"I think you can safely take the handcuffs off him," the FBI man said, then his hand reached out to something off screen and the connection was broken.

The younger DEA agent nodded to the other one, who motioned for the doctor to lean forward. Carras was sitting in what would have normally been the boss agent's chair so that he could be seen by the mini-camera clipped to the monitor. There was a click and then another, and Carras's hands were free. He brought his hands in front of him and massaged his aching forearms, then worked his shoulders to loosen them. The pain slid down the scale from sharp to dull. "Satisfied?" he said.

"Sorry," the balding agent said. Carras wondered if anything he said ever matched the tone in which he said it.

"So now what?" the doctor said.

The agent was the DEA's senior representative on the anti-trafficking task force. He spread his hands, palms up and said, "So now, nothing." He switched off the monitor and indicated the door. "You're free to go."

Carras stood up. He was dressed in odds and ends from the hospital's lost and found, including flip-flop slippers that were a little too large. "That's it?" he said.

"What do you want from us?" said the DEA man. He gestured for Carras to move away from his chair so he could sit down at the desk.

Carras wasn't budging. "I want some clothes and a plane ticket home."

"We're not the Red Cross. Now, you want to move, I got work to do."

Carras picked up the phone and when the balding man moved his hand as if to prevent him he said, "So far you've just been doing your job, and it's too bad I'm not the criminal mastermind you wanted me to be. But in the past three days I've been kidnaped, worked like a slave, and forced to risk my life to escape, and I'm all out of patience. The least you're going to do is let me make a phone call then give me a ride over to a hotel."

"Or what?" the agent said.

Carras said, "I have performed life-saving procedures on two senators, five congressmen and four former cabinet secretaries. And if you don't back off right now I will do my damnedest to sic every last one of them on you," he turned the nameplate on the agent's desk and read out the name, "Agent Warren P. Hennenfent."

After a moment, Agent Warren P. Hennenfent replied that it would be his pleasure to let Carras use his telephone. Again, his tone did not match the substance of the message, but Carras didn't care.

An hour later the doctor was soaking in a tub in a suite at the best hotel in Grand Caicos. The hot water leached some of the pain from his back and shoulders, but the bump on his head was taking its own time about going down.

When he got out of the bath there was a fleecy terry-cloth robe to wear, then a man summoned by the concierge brought over a selection of suits, shirts and the necessities that Carras would need before he stepped onto an airplane, including shoes. He tried things on until he had what he needed then signed a chit that would add the cost to his hotel bill.

It had all been arranged through one phone call to Charlie Vance on the DEA agent's phone. His friend had been surprised to hear that Carras was in the Turks and Caicos; Vance had thought that he was on Amtrak heading west to meet Costas. But he got over the shock of hearing Carras's nutshell summary of what had happened since their last meeting and swung into action. He'd arranged through his travel agent for the hotel, clothes and a plane ticket home, and he'd tugged strings to make sure the US consulate issued Carras a temporary proof of citizenship to get him through airport security.

"You're a good friend, Charlie," Carras had said when Vance told him he would take care of everything.

There was a silence on the line. "You sure you're all right, Ath?" Vance said. "You don't sound the same."

"I'm just tired," Carras said. "And I need to get this thing over with and move on."

• • •

The FBI's Connecticut field office was on an upper floor of the federal building at 600 State Street in New Haven and had a good view of the harbor but Carras and Charlie Vance were ignoring the vista while they focused on the man sitting at the desk between them and the corner office window. Special Agent in Charge Richard Fillmore was giving them the kind of tepidness they might have expected from a undergraduate who hadn't prepared a term paper and was looking for a good excuse.

"The problem is, we've got absolutely no evidence that a crime has been committed," the special agent said.

"Dr. Carras crashed a stolen plane—stolen from drug smugglers—onto a Caribbean island," Vance said. "He was wearing nothing but a burlap sack. Are you saying that doesn't indicate to you that something out of the ordinary was going on?"

Fillmore's snowy white French cuffs were held together by cufflinks made from gold coins. He shot them now so that they caught the sunlight that lay across his orderly desk top. "Of course it does," he said. "But apart from Dr. Carras's information, there is no indication that a criminal act has taken place on US soil. No signs of a struggle at the apartment. No fingerprints. No

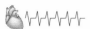

witnesses. No ransom note or phone calls. And the two men he has accused of putting him in the trunk of a car have credible alibis—not to mention the fact that they are reputable businessmen with no criminal records or known associations."

There was more of it but none of it was helpful to Athan Carras. The Bureau had his complaint on file. Evidence technicians had gone through his apartment and found everything normal, his wallet, keys and cell phone neatly arranged on his bedside table. Leonard Maigrot and Isaac Dumoulin had been interviewed, in the presence of heavyweight legal representation, and had denied every allegation of wrong-doing.

Fillmore leafed through a file on his desk and asked Carras, "Did you ever approach the Flynnt Group for funding for an experiment in..." he placed a finger on the page, "is this right?—suspended animation?"

"It's called deep hypothermic circulatory arrest," said Carras. "And, no, I did not ask the Flynnt Group for funding."

"Did you go to Mr. Flynnt's residence in the Bahamas without an invitation and badger him about a grant?"

"I was invited by a guest of Mr. Flynnt. And the substance of our conversation is in the information I filed with this office a week ago. I did not ask Flynnt for anything. He asked me to perform a heart transplant on his son on his yacht."

"On his yacht?" Fillmore said. "You're sure of that?"

"I saw the operating room."

"Did you get into a fistfight with a reporter in Miami?"

"What? Of course not."

"I see." Fillmore closed the file. "Well, you can understand, doctor, that we have some... dissonance here."

Vance spoke up. "That's because somebody's gone to a lot of trouble to make it look that way."

"Or perhaps your friend likes being written up in the newspapers and interviewed on TV talk shows. There was a lot of that not so long ago."

"Are you accusing me of being a publicity hound?" Carras said.

Fillmore's shrug involved only one shoulder but it was as dismissive as if he had used both. "You wouldn't be the first academic to have his head turned by a little media attention."

"That's ridiculous!"

"Maybe," Fillmore said. "All I know is, you're here now, safe and sound except for a bump on your head. Perhaps this has all been some kind of misunderstanding."

"You've got to be kidding," Carras said. He started to rise but Vance put a restraining hand on his arm.

"Come on," his friend said. "We're not doing any good here."

In the elevator on the way down, Vance said, "They've been got at."

"By whom?" Carras said. "Who's got enough clout to get at the FBI?"

"That's the problem," Vance said. "It's a short list and very exclusive. It's also way out of our reach."

As Vance drove them back to the campus, Carras said, "The funny thing is, I'm not all that angry about it any more. I almost feel that I owe Terry Flynnt for giving me a challenge when I needed one."

"Do you feel like you owe him enough to cut some poor bastard's heart out and put it in his son's chest?"

"No," said Carras, "and that's the problem. There's no guarantee Flynnt's willing to call it a draw."

"So how do we stop him from trying again?"

Carras had already thought about it. "Philip," he said at last. "And Annabella. They're the only ones close to him who aren't under his control."

They were pulling into Vance's parking spot at the Sterling Hall of Medicine. "Okay," he said, "let's call them up."

Carras shook his head as he undid the seat belt. "We'd never get their number. And if we did, we wouldn't get them on the phone. Too many layers of security."

Whenever Vance was thinking hard he looked even more like Jack Nicholson. "We can't reach them, but we know where they are," he said. "And I have a plane."

"We don't know where they are," Carras said, "All we know is that it's one island among several hundred in the Bahamas and it's almost certainly well guarded by men with guns. I don't recall ever hearing the name of the place."

"First things first," Vance said, his eyebrows working like a semaphore. "To the Internet." He led the way to his office and the computer on his desk. But no search engine had a listing under "Terry Flynnt, island, Bahamas."

"Damn," Vance said. "Who do we know who would know?"

"Nobody," Carras said, then corrected himself. "Hilary Cartiere."

"Call her," Vance said, turning the desk phone toward Carras.

"I already tried that. I got no farther than her agent's receptionist."

"Let's see how I do," Vance said.

• • •

Isaac Dumoulin was in the Boeing jet flying west. The cabin attendant had been sent forward and he was on a scrambled phone connection to Terry Flynnt.

"I'm asking you, are you still sure you want to do this? There are other surgeons."

Flynnt's voice, digitalized, randomized and reconstituted, had lost none of its flat toned certainty. "He's the one I want. Everything he's done shows that he's the kind who gets it done."

"You got that right," Isaac said.

"Like you and me," Flynnt said.

"But not like Maigrot. I'm worried about him."

"Maigrot's nothing. He'll do as he's told."

"Still, I worry," Isaac said.

"That's the nature of your job. Let me know when it's done. I'll see you on the boat." Flynnt cut the connection.

• • •

"Sid Hoffman's office," said his secretary in a stiff British accent.

The voice on the phone said, "This is Jack Nicholson. Is Sid around?"

"I'm sorry, Mr. Nicholson. He's in Palm Springs. May I have him call you?"

"Nah. Listen, I'm here with Norman Jewison and we're looking at a project that might be just right for Hilary Cartiere."

"I'm sure Mr. Hoffman would be delighted to set something up."

"Right. In the meantime, can you give me Hilary's number? I don't think it ever made it from the Rolodex to the Palm Pilot."

"I'm sorry, Mr. Nicholson, I'm not at liberty..."

"Look, sweetie, I guarantee you we're not going to talk deal. We just want to know if she'd be interested. We were thinking Faye Dunaway and we can always go back there."

Sid Hoffman did not handle Faye Dunaway, his secretary was well aware. She also knew that she was never more than one bad decision away from the unemployment line. Pissing off Jack Nicholson and Norman Jewison while losing a part for Hilary Cartiere could be bad enough to shoot her right past the queue and onto a plane back to the musty old flat in Hammersmith. She said, "It's area code 310," and read out the number.

"Thank you, darling," said Charlie Vance in his best Nicholson ever.

• • •

Hilary Cartiere was by the pool behind the house in Bel-Air that she bought after *A Thousand Ships*. The pool's kidney shape was no longer fashionable and the grouting needed work, but those failings did not trouble her now the way they had only three weeks before. She was sipping iced tea and leafing through the one of the stack of scripts Sid had sent over. There was a good part in this one—of course, it would need substantial rewrite, definitely more lines for her character—and she was already trying out one of the speeches.

The maid brought out the phone. "Señora, Meester Jack Neecholson," she said.

"Jack, darling, it's been ages."

"It's Athan Carras," said the voice on the phone. "Sorry for the pretense, but I guess that makes us even."

"How'd you get this number?" Hilary said.

"Never mind. And don't hang up or your next caller will be from the National Inquirer wanting to know what it's like to hire yourself out to crazy billionaires."

The California sun seemed to lose some of its candlepower. "What do you want?" Hilary said.

"The name of the island we were on."

"I don't know it."

"Listen, Hilary, I'm not blaming you for anything. Flynnt's not a guy who's easy to turn down and you did what you had to do. Fact is, you gave me one of the most memorable nights of my life, and it's my fault if I didn't let myself see that I was being suckered."

"It wasn't all pretense," Hilary said. "You were very sweet."

"It doesn't matter now."

"I honestly can't help you."

"Look, Hilary," said Carras. "This is not about my wounded ego. Let me lay it out for you. Terry Flynnt wants me to cut the heart out of a bought-and-paid-for donor to save his son's life. That's murder and I'm not going to do it."

Murder? Hilary Cartiere didn't want anything to do with this. "That's awful, just awful," she said. She remembered how she'd said the exact line in *Now and Forever* and gave it precisely the same punch. She hadn't lost any of the old power.

"I'm going to fly down to see Philip and Annabella," Carras was saying. "They're the only ones who can stop Flynnt. All I need from you is the name of the island. I'll do the rest."

"I'm so sorry."

"Hilary, let me be clear about this. After I left the island, the man kidnaped me and put me through hell. I almost died. I'm not going to let it happen again. If you help me solve this quietly this is the last you'll ever hear about it."

"And if I don't?"

"Then expect that call from the Inquirer."

Somewhere inside Hilary Cartiere there remained a remnant of Hilda McCarty, the small town girl who believed in uncomplicated love and happy endings and who had walked a few yards along a beach with Athan Carras. She might have come out again, but Hilary had long ago learned to separate her emotions from her business. Now she thought the situation through with cold calculation.

Publicity, even the scurrilous mud-slinging of the tabloids, wouldn't do her any real harm. As Sam Goldwyn was supposed to have said, Publicity is good. Good publicity is even better. But if bad publicity made Flynnt reneg on the guarantee of financing for her comeback picture, it wouldn't be long before Hilary Cartiere was playing Sunset Boulevard's Norah Desmond without the camera.

You swear you won't mention my name?" she said.

"I swear."

"It's called Forlorn Island."

"Thank you."

"Athan," she said, "you're a nice man. I wish... never mind. Don't call me again."

• • •

"We can fly down to Miami by tonight then go out to the island first thing in the morning," Vance said. "Catch them early."

"This could be dangerous, Charlie. You don't know Flynnt."

Vance laughed. "My father told me never to advertise it, but we come from similar stock. My grandfather and his brothers made their money as rum runners during Prohibition. Believe me, I know the breed."

Carras struck his forehead with the heel of his hand. "Damn," he said. "I haven't called Costas. He'll be expecting me to show up in the Pantera." He reached for his cell phone and entered Beth's number. There was no answer.

• • •

Leonard Maigrot told his assistant not to put through any calls except those from Isaac and Flynnt. He turned his plush, leather-covered chair toward the window and sat slumped as he watched the work down in the gray scar where the twin towers had been. There was a lesson there, he thought, a lesson that maybe didn't apply to the likes of Terry Flynnt but it certainly applied to ordinary mortals who ascended to the heights where the truly rich flew: you could be way up there in the clear air above the world but you could come crashing down in no time at all.

The visit from the FBI agents had scared Maigrot, even though Isaac had told him that a fix was in at the highest levels. Flynnt himself had made the call. But Maigrot was so rattled that he made the mistake of letting the security chief see his distress. After that, he was out of the loop. Now, whatever was going on, the ball was still in play, but Maigrot was no longer part of it. And that worried him.

It had to be personal for Flynnt, he thought; that was the only way it made sense. The continuing pursuit was purely ego-driven. Maigrot had nothing against egotism, but he'd swung long enough through the upper-most treetops of the corporate jungle to know that there was a line between commonplace arrogance and the outrageous cancer of pride that could blind a man like Terry Flynnt to the long fall that awaited even the truly rich who tried to leap too far.

But if Maigrot's world was collapsing beneath him, he wouldn't know until it was too late. It was all between Flynnt and Isaac now. Not for the first time, Maigrot wondered what the link was between these two men who should have been almost separate species, the son of a bigoted Irish immigrant and a fatherless product of a Midwest black ghetto.

Maigrot had long since researched Isaac Dumoulin—at least he had gathered what little intelligence he could find. As a kid, Isaac had a job sweeping up in the Flynnt plastics factory in a rundown industrial park outside Cleveland, back when Terry Flynnt was earning a chemical engineering degree from the University of Chicago. Not long after the younger Flynnt returned, his father had died in a fall at the plant—drunk, the police report said. About the same time, Isaac had enlisted in the Army.

A few years passed, Terry Flynnt developed his first patented product with a military application, and he apparently reached out to bring Captain Dumoulin into the business. They had been inseparable ever since. Maigrot had seen corporate ladder climbers try to insinuate themselves between the chairman of the Flynnt Group and his director of security. They tried to undercut Isaac and steal some of the light that came to him through his closeness to the pinnacle. The intriguers had soon found themselves riding the longest snake in the game, all the way down to oblivion.

Maigrot had never made that mistake. He had stepped carefully around Isaac Dumoulin, had deferred to the man's judgment and never put himself in the position where Flynnt would have to choose between them.

But there were other ways to blow it at this level of the game. One way was to be the designated fall guy. Flynnt had fixed the last disaster by making a phone call, but even the kind of money Flynnt donated to presidential and congressional campaigns didn't allow him to make such calls whenever he screwed the pooch. And they'd been lucky: If Carras had been dead when he was pulled out of the plane wreck, somebody might have kept on asking questions until some uncomfortable answers began to turn up.

Maigrot had to face the bowel-chilling prospect that if his boss had gone totally, unrestrainedly, Howard Hughes crazy, he would keep pushing the Carras situation until it went far beyond any hope of containment. A multibillionaire with an obsession could make a hell of a mess. And, unfortunately, this mess would have Leonard Maigrot's fingerprints on every flat surface. If somebody had to stand beneath a shower of shit, he was the obvious choice.

It was probably time to make a move. If he knew for certain that Flynnt and Isaac were pushing the doctor again, right now, there would be no question. If they weren't ready to cut their losses and walk, Leonard Maigrot was.

His intercom buzzed and he swung the chair around to face the desk. His wish—that it would be Isaac calling to tell him Flynnt wanted him to find another doctor—would have been a prayer if Maigrot had not long ago switched from God to Mammon. But his assistant said, "I'm sorry to bother you, sir, but it's Ms. Cartiere. She's called three times and says it's very urgent."

"Tell her I'm in a meeting."

"I did. She says to tell you it's about the doctor."

Maigrot pushed the flashing button on his phone. "Leonard Maigrot," he said.

"Carras phoned me," Hilary said. "I think he's gone crazy."

"Tell me what he said."

"First we need to talk about our deal."

Maigrot needed to hear what Carras was saying, but he kept the anger out of his voice. "There's nothing to talk about there. You did what you contracted to do and we're living up to our side of it. The agreed upon line of credit has been set aside to guarantee a picture of your choice."

"Well, that's just not going to do anymore," the actress said. "The pot just got a lot richer."

"I don't know what you're talking about."

"Carras told me what Flynnt wants him to do."

Now it was time to be very cool. Maigrot said, "I don't see how that makes a difference."

Hilary Cartiere could be even cooler. "You will when you hear what it is."

In a negotiation, Maigrot knew, the smartest reply to that kind of tease was no reply. But he had a strong feeling that what the woman was about to tell him would make even more of a difference to him than she thought it would. "All right," he said, "what do you want?"

"I want the Full Lucy," she said.

"The what?"

"I want what Lucille Ball had, full control of an independent production studio."

"I have no idea what that means," Maigrot said. "I'm not saying that as a negotiating posture. I just don't know what it entails."

She spelled it out for him. She wanted the original financing guarantee for her comeback picture, but she wanted it amplified and extended to three other pictures, plus she wanted backing for two television pilots a year for four years, with an option to renew the terms of the deal at her discretion.

"That's one hell of a blank check," Maigrot told her.

"You're still the primary preferred investor," she said. "You get the first money out and most of the back end."

"If there's any money out. If there's any back end."

"Well, that's why they call it risk capital."

In a real negotiation, Maigrot would have stalled and haggled. But what the hell, he thought. "Okay, you've got it. Now what did the doctor say?"

But Hilary Cartiere wasn't ready to work on a handshake. She had a deal memo already drafted. "I'll fax it to you for signature," she said. "Or if you have an electronic signature set-up, I'll e-mail it to you."

The Flynnt Group was up to date on communications technology. Maigrot lit up his work station and told her to e-mail the document. It was on his monitor in seconds. He scanned it then went through the simple routine that affixed his signature on behalf of the corporation and automatically filed it with the company's legal department and Hilary Cartiere's lawyer and agent. "Done," he said. "Now what did the doctor say?"

He listened in growing horror as she told him. The dread was not occasioned by the nastiness of what Carras had said: that Flynnt wanted to take the heart of a third world donor and put it in Philip Flynnt's chest. Maigrot was a firm believer in the marketplace, and if people wanted to sell their organs, even their lives, it was nobody's business but that of the parties to the transaction.

What horrified him was the knowledge that Flynnt's control of the Flynnt Group was even more precarious than Maigrot had lately begun to fear. He hadn't known—no one had known—that Philip Flynnt was near death and that his substantial holdings in the corporation might soon be on the open market.

With all the stock Terry Flynnt had been selling to raise the pool of capital he'd intended for the research foundation, the old man might already have effectively lost control of the company. The next directors' meeting could see a coup by Victor Whitehall. If Whitehall had bought up enough Flynnt Group stock since the last meeting of the board—*my God, what if he heard about the private placements and bought one or more of them?*—he had only to shake the board's tree and the fruits would fall into his lap.

Hilary Cartiere was still talking but Maigrot had missed the last part. "Say that again," he said.

"Carras is going down to the island," she said. "He thinks that Philip can stop his father."

"When will he get there?"

"Who knows? But I think he's on his way right now."

"Is that it," Maigrot said. "Is that all of it?"

"If Philip can't help, he's thinking about going to the tabloids."

"Okay," Maigrot said. "Is that all of it?"

"That's not enough?" she said.

He made a throat sound that could have meant anything and hung up the phone. Maigrot knew what the sound meant: it was the sound Julius Caesar must have made when he came to whatever that Roman river was and knew that he had to lead his army over it. It was the going-for-broke sound.

At least he wouldn't have to worry about the ridiculous deal he had made with Hilary Cartiere. The Full Lucy, she'd called it. Well, good luck to her when she tried to get the new owners of the Flynnt Group to honor it.

He turned and watched for a while the big machines down in the scar where the World Trade Towers used to stand. Then he picked up the phone, opened his private, secure line and punched in the number he'd memorized after the FBI men had left.

• • •

Victor Whitehall was in conference with his key people. It was not a happy session for one of them: The ex-CIA man Fletcher had nothing new on the Flynnt Group and was trying to cloud his situation report with what he called "informed speculation." That kind of bunkum used to work at least some of the time back at Langley, but Whitehall could see through Fletcher's clouds as if he had been born with Doppler radar.

"Bullshit," the old man said. "You got nothing, and I'm getting fed up paying for nothing."

"We could send in Larkin," Fletcher said.

Whitehall thought about it. By purchasing on the market and by collaring Flynnt's supposedly private placements, he had assembled sufficient stock to press for a second seat on the Flynnt Group board. But two seats were not enough; Terry and Philip Flynnt still controlled more shares than any other director and the older Flynnt's personality still dominated the board. Whitehall needed a lever, some issue that would weaken Flynnt's authority and swing the fund managers over to his camp. The retired major general would go whichever way the wind blew, and Whitehall would control the company.

Whitehall knew that victory in a struggle like this was in the timing. You had to know when to push and then you pushed hard. Was it time to push now, time to push it all the way?

"How would Larkin do it?" he said.

"A small rubber inflatable with a silenced motor, swim the last two miles underwater in scuba gear," Fletcher said. "Flynnt does business almost exclusively from the yacht these days. Larkin goes aboard, gets all the information he can, brings it back or sends it out by modem."

Whitehall looked at the others around the table, saw their carefully attentive but uncommitted expressions. Not one of them was going to approve or condemn Fletcher's plan until they saw which way the boss was leaning. *Fucking brown-nosers,* he thought. They were nothing, and they'd be less than nothing without men like him. And men like Flynnt.

His private line rang and he almost let his underlings see that he was startled. Most of the handful of people who knew that number were in this room, and he wasn't expecting to hear from the ones who weren't.

He reached for the phone and said, "Whitehall." A moment later he said, "Who is this?"

Each of his advisers looked in a different direction, none of them at him. Whitehall listened to the voice on the phone and said, "I may be interested. What do you want for that information?" He listened a few seconds more then he said, "Agreed. But not over the phone. Come to my office now."

He hung up and sat for a moment with his hands palm down on the desk, face immobile. Then his small black eyes flicked to Arthur Pennock, his director on the Flynnt Group board. "Call the other Flynnt directors," he said, "but not the Flynnts. Warn them that you might be about to convene an emergency meeting of the board by conference call. Grave and urgent business that could crash the share value. Advise them not to discuss the matter with anyone—especially not with Terry Flynnt—until they hear from you."

To Fletcher he said, "Get Larkin on deck. But we're not going in surreptitiously. We're going in bold, right through the front door. We've got Flynnt by the balls and we're going to squeeze the juice out of him."

• • •

In his corner office, Leonard Maigrot's hand shook so badly that his phone's handset rattled against its cradle as he hung up. He looked out again at all the empty space between him and the unforgiving pavement down below. He had made his leap, was in the air, and would land either soft or hard.

Terry Flynnt made a bad enemy. If he fought off Whitehall and remained in control of the company, the least he would do would be to end Leonard Maigrot's business career. And if what Maigrot suspected about some of Isaac's "security operations" was true, the stakes would be higher than a top-floor corner office. Maigrot would be playing for his life.

But if Whitehall won, and if Maigrot's defection was the key to that victory, then the reward could be everything Leonard Maigrot had ever wanted.

He looked around his office. There was nothing here he wanted to take with him. He went out and told his assistant he would be gone for a while then stepped into the express elevator. He felt his stomach lurch upwards as he plunged toward his future.

Chapter 14

The twin engined Piper was a little more than an hour west of Miami when Charlie Vance said, "That should be it."

The green and white smear on the northeast horizon grew clearer as they approached at five thousand feet. In a few minutes, they could make out the hill with its glass walled residence glinting in the morning sun and then the paved airstrip running most of the island's length. Flynnt's vast yacht was still tied up at the dock on the island's west side.

"You know," said Vance, "I think this is the first time we've flown together that you don't seem nervous."

"I guess I'm focused on what's going to happen after we land," said Carras.

"Funny thing is, the prospect of being met by armed guards working for a guy who's not afraid to order a kidnaping gives me the collywobbles."

Carras rubbed his hands together. "I just want to get this over with."

"You ask me, you're looking forward to it," Vance said, then he stopped and listened to his earphones for a moment and said, "Here we go."

Vance touched a control on the instrument panel and through his own earphones Carras heard, "...any unauthorized landing will be met with armed response. Veer off now and leave the area. Repeat, inbound Piper aircraft.

You are approaching a private airstrip. You are not authorized to land and any unauthorized..."

Vance toggled a switch and said, "This is Piper Chief Bravo Four One Niner Six. I am out of fuel and request permission for an emergency landing."

"Permission denied," said the voice, "Veer off."

"No can do," said Vance. "You want to shoot me down it's about the same as crashing into the sea. But you'll have to explain it to Bahamian air traffic control."

There was a silence then the voice said, "Do not leave the plane after touchdown. I repeat, any attempt to do so will be met by armed response."

"Roger," said Vance and signed off. "This is it," he said to Carras and turned the plane on its left wing.

There were four of them, dressed in lightweight khaki uniforms and climbing out of a jeep as the Piper rolled to a stop and Vance cut the engine. Three of them carried automatic rifles and the fourth had a pistol holstered on his belt. As the propeller wound down to a stop, they surrounded the plane, weapons leveled at the occupants. The pistol wearer approached Carras's side and took off his mirror-lensed sunglasses to inspect both doctors. A label on his shirt pocket read Frankl.

"Stay where you are," he said. "We'll refuel you and get you out of here."

Carras slid the window open. "We lied," he said. "We're not out of fuel."

The man drew his pistol and pointed it at Carras. His thumb pulled back the hammer. "Turn this around and get out of here now. Do anything else and I'll shoot to kill."

The other men were aiming their rifles now, fingers on triggers. Carras said, "This is family business. Flynnt family business." It was a stratagem Vance and he had agreed on. "You better call it in."

Without lowering the pistol Frankl stepped back and spoke into a small radio mike clipped to the epaulet of his shirt. The response came via an earphone and after he heard it he said to Carras, "Who are you?"

Carras identified himself and the man relayed the information. They all waited for the reply, the seconds stretching past a minute while the muzzles of the guns remained pointed at the men in the plane. Then the man put his sunglasses back on and said, "Out of the plane. Slowly, and show your hands."

The two doctors stood with their palms against the fuselage and their feet wide apart while the man with the pistol frisked them thoroughly. Then they were crowded into the back of the jeep. They headed to the main road but when the vehicle swung west instead of toward the hill, Carras said, "Take me to the house. I'm here to see Philip Flynnt."

Frankl turned and said, "Mr. Philip is on the yacht. And Mr. Flynnt says to tell you, 'You're expected.'"

The jeep delivered them to the end of the jetty. The man with the sunglasses indicated the gangplank but made no move to accompany them.

Isaac Dumoulin was waiting at the top of the ramp. He smiled a small, tight smile. "Welcome back, doctor," he said. "You saved us having to send the jet for you."

"You were sure I would come?" Carras said.

"Mr. Flynnt was." Isaac looked Vance up and down then raised his eyebrows.

Vance introduced himself and offered his hand. Isaac took it. The smile got a tiny fraction wider as the security chief said, "We may already have all the doctors we need. Are you another heart specialist?"

Vance shook his head. "Medical ethics."

Isaac looked at Carras. "Did you think we were going to have a debate?"

Carras said, "I want to see Philip."

"He's not available right now."

"I want to see him."

"He's sleeping. Gupta gave him a sedative."

"Then I want to see Annabella."

"She was a little upset. He gave her something to calm her down. She's resting in the house."

"Then I'd better see Flynnt."

Isaac lost the smile. "Well, that's what you came for, isn't it? He's in the lounge." The security chief turned to Vance and said, "You'd better come, too. We may need an ethics counselor after all."

Flynnt was grinding away on the Lifecycle 800 when Isaac led the two doctors into the room. He made a perfunctory introduction of Charlie Vance then stood with his back to the door they had entered through, powerful hands clasped before him.

Carras crossed the wide room to the lean figure on the cycle and said, "Flynnt, we have to end this."

"We are ending it, doctor. The rest of the medical team flew in this morning."

"I'm not doing the operation."

Flynnt didn't stop pedaling. "Yes, you are."

"I won't kill anybody, even somebody who thinks he's willing to die," Carras said. "Not so you can hold on to what you've got."

The old man stopped pedaling and looked at Carras as if he was the most curious specimen he had ever seen. "You're a gifted surgeon, doctor," he said. "And you've turned out to be a lot tougher than I thought you were. But, by god, I've known street sweepers who have more insight into the human heart."

"What do you mean?" Carras said but before Flynnt could reply the phone beside the cycle beeped and the old man answered it. As he listened, his face hardened. He thanked the caller and hung up then turned to Isaac and said, "That was a friend of ours in the Royal Bahamas Police Force. An RBPF helicopter is on its way from Nassau. It could be here any moment."

"I'll get the rest of the med team on board right away," Isaac said.

"No," said Flynnt. "No time. We need to be in international waters asap." He called the yacht's captain on the intercom and said, "Get us out to sea, all possible speed. And maintain complete radio silence."

"We're not going with you," Carras said. He felt a vibration through the carpeting under his feet. The yacht's diesels were turning over. "Let us off," he said.

"Too late now, doctor," Flynnt said. To Isaac he said, "Tell Frankl the crew on shore is to cooperate fully with the Bahamians—so fully that it takes them ten times longer than normal to do anything."

"Got it," Isaac said.

"What's going on?" Carras said.

"Nothing to do with you, doctor," Flynnt said. "Why don't you go down to the operating room and get scrubbed up? Your friend too. He can assist."

Carras crossed his arms. "I told you, I will not kill for you. I'd rather die myself than take a life."

Flynnt laughed, a sound without humor, and picked up his phone again. "You mean you'd rather die than lose. But what makes you think that's the choice you'll be offered? Isaac, take them down."

The security chief produced an efficient-looking automatic pistol.

"I can't operate on Philip if you shoot me," Carras said.

"Depends on where I shoot you," Isaac said.

Vance said, "I think he means it, Ath."

As they left the room, Flynnt was on the phone again. "Get me our contact in the Ministry of National Security in the Government of the Bahamas."

● ● ●

Victor Whitehall was not impressed by Leonard Maigrot. All brains and no balls was his assessment, but he brought him along on the trip down to Nassau. He wished he'd been able to win over Isaac Dumoulin, or even find a man of equivalent ability that he could trust the way Flynnt trusted his chief of security. But such men were rare.

Whitehall had researched Dumoulin more thoroughly than Maigrot had but even his best investigators hadn't cracked the enigma of the bond between Dumoulin and Flynnt. The head of the industrial intelligence firm who prepared the written dossier had a more literary style than most of his kind and used the word "mystery" advisedly. "There is a secret at the heart of the relationship, and only the two of them know what it is," the report said.

It had something to do with the death years ago of Roddy Flynnt, Terry's father, who had been found dying at the foot of the flight of stairs that led up to his office in the plastics factory. Terry himself had done the finding two hours after the factory closed. He had been working in the small research lab he had built behind the main building. He called an ambulance but the old man was DOA at the emergency room of Case Western Reserve University Hospital.

The coroner ruled it death by misadventure: Roddy Flynnt was known to favor drinking by himself in the office after the place closed for the day—there was only one shift back then—and his blood alcohol level was well up.

The investigator dug up rumors that there had been an "incident" involving one of the young women who worked on the shop floor. The boss was also periodically known to call a factory girl—black or white, pretty or plain—up to the office to find out how much she wanted to keep her job. The price of steady employment involved applying various parts of her anatomy to Roddy Flynnt's.

The girl's name had been Urlene Cuddiford. She was now Mrs. Urlene Sharpe. Interviewed by an investigator who pretended to be a Cleveland cop working on a "cold squad" that closed old open cases, she professed to remember nothing of the alleged incident. The report said it was likely that the old drunk had been chasing the girl and had fallen down the stairs. She may even have pushed him to get his hands off her and left him dying.

None of that explained Terry Flynnt and Isaac Dumoulin. The one interesting wrinkle was that Dumoulin had presented himself at a US Army recruiting center that same afternoon as a volunteer. If there was a connection between the two events, the investigator couldn't make it. Terry Flynnt swore at the coroner's inquest that the then eighteen-year-old Dumoulin had left at the end of the shift and that the younger Flynnt had seen him go before he locked up the factory and went out to the lab.

If there had been any relationship between Isaac Dumoulin and Urlene Cuddiford, nobody had talked about it then and nobody was talking about it now.

"There's the police copter," Leonard Maigrot said, breaking Whitehall's chain of thought. The black and white machine was coming in from behind them, passing almost directly over the heads of Whitehall and his party in the small, fast boat provided by Larkin, the bare-skulled ex-SBS commando who was at the wheel. They were less than two miles east of Forlorn Island.

"The timing's good," Maigrot said. "We can run right up onto the beach while Dumoulin's busy dealing with the cops."

Whitehall didn't like men who made a habit of belaboring the obvious. In return for Maigrot's defection, he had promised to place the turncoat in charge of one of the Flynnt Group business divisions once control had passed to the new ownership. He was leaning toward not keeping that promise.

"The yacht's moored on the other side," Maigrot said. "We can get a vehicle at the hangar and cut right across."

Whitehall decided that the man had a tendency to chatter when nervous. The old man thought briefly of having Larkin break his neck and throw him over the side, just to shut him up. But the chatterbox might still be useful.

• • •

Philip Flynnt was on table two in the operating room under green sterile drapes. The Guptas were with him: the female half of the pair was injecting something into the IV that connected to the patient's arm; the Indian doctor was laying out the tubing from the heart-lung machine. He looked up when he saw Carras watching him through the door's round window, then went quickly back to what he was doing.

A few moments later, Gupta nudged open the door with his toe, keeping his gloved hands up. "It is an honor to be working with you, doctor," he said. "I hope you will not judge us too harshly."

Carras said, "You'll have to answer to your own conscience, doctor. I have no intention of performing an operation here."

The other's brown eyes widened above his mask, but whatever he was about to say was cut off by the arrival of Flynnt.

"With me," the billionaire said, motioning Carras and Vance to accompany him down a short hallway and into a small cabin that contained a hospital bed and was fitted out as a post-op recovery room. There was only one chair and the old man took it, leaving the two doctors to stand, Carras thought, like schoolboys called to the principal's office.

"There isn't much time," Flynnt said, "and I need to set something straight."

"I'm tired of this game," Carras said. "You seem to have a pathological need to make everything a contest where the winner has to be you. I refuse to play."

"You think this is a game?" Flynnt said. "God help us, man. You know, doctor, I chose you for your hands and your brain. They're the best and I will have the best for my son. But you've got to be the biggest walking irony I've ever come across—a heart doctor who knows everything about the human heart except how it feels to have one."

"Wait just a minute," Carras began but the old man cut him off.

"I don't have a minute to spare for you. My son is dying and you are going to save him." He turned to Vance, "You're not by any chance a Catholic are you, doctor?"

Vance said, "Sorry. Episcopalian to the core."

"But you are a moral man?"

"I've devoted my life to the study of ethics, of right and wrong. It's taught me that each often interpenetrates the other and all we can do is to try to do as much good as we can while we're here."

"You think God judges us on our intentions, even when our efforts don't measure up?"

"He'd better."

Flynnt rubbed a hand across his face. For the first time, Carras noticed the liver spots of age; for the first time, too, he saw the tired and elderly man who lived behind the hard facade Terry Flynnt normally showed the world.

"I wish I'd thought to bring a priest," Flynnt said. "What the Church says about 'as the twig is bent' is true. If they get you early in life, it doesn't matter if they lose you for most of the middle. They'll get you back again at the end."

"I don't understand," Carras said.

"I think I do," Vance said. "You feel the need to confess."

"I do," said Flynnt. "I have a sin that weighs on my soul, an old sin and a terrible one. Tell me, doctor of ethics, if a man killed his father would God punish him by taking his son?"

"No," said Vance. "God does not punish the innocent with the guilty."

"You killed your father?" Carras said.

"Near as," said Flynnt. And now he let the hardness drop so that a great sadness took control of the old man's face, drawing out its length and filling his eyes with a luster that made Carras think of the gold flecked icons of sad eyed martyrs that hung in the Greek church his parents had taken him to as a boy.

The billionaire knelt on the carpet and clasped his hands before him, staring straight ahead. "He was a bugger, my old man," he said. "Never saw a bottle he didn't leave empty or a good looking woman he didn't have a go at. He was a devil for the girls who worked in the factory. One night he tried it on with the little black girl that Isaac was sweet on, but he didn't know that Isaac was waiting for her at the door to walk her home.

"She screamed and Isaac came running. The girl ran out of the office at the top of the stairs with my dad right after her, laughing and half-drunk, though half-drunk for him meant he'd taken enough drink to lay most men out cold.

"The girl ran down the stairs as Isaac came up. He took my father and threw him down the steps and when the old man got to the bottom he wasn't moving."

Flynnt's eyes were unfocused now, not seeing the two men in the room with him, only the silent factory and the scene on the stairs. "I saw it happen," he said. "I told Isaac he'd have to go. He'd been talking about the army and I said, 'Go now and sign up, get away from this.' The girl was out the door and gone, she hadn't seen what happened. It was just me and him and Isaac didn't deserve what they would have done to him, a young black boy who'd attacked a white man."

Vance said, "But he didn't kill him, did he?"

Flynnt's voice came from far away, from a distance of almost forty years. He said, "No, that was me. I had to give Isaac time to get down to the recruiting office. So I sat beside my father until I thought it was long enough, two hours maybe, then I called the ambulance and told them I'd just found him. If I'd called right away, I think they could have saved him."

His eyes came back into focus now and he looked up at Vance. "He'd done enough harm. What was the point in letting him destroy Isaac's life? He would have done it. He was a great one for vengeance and the settling of scores."

Vance said, "I'm not a priest but I was raised Catholic. I know the rules. Do you sincerely repent of the sin you've confessed?"

"I do, before God," Flynnt said.

"And have you performed an appropriate act of contrition?"

"I have given my son the freedom I never had, so he could make a happy life for himself. And I have been a brother to Isaac."

Vance put his hand on the old man's head and said, "Then I would say you have brought good out of evil, which is what God asks of us. If I were a priest I would absolve you and let you die free from this weight on your soul."

Flynnt crossed himself and stood up. "Thank you," he said to Vance.

"I don't understand," Carras said. "You're not liable to die for years yet."

Vance put his arm around his friend's shoulders and said, "You know, Ath, I think the man is right. You may be the most brilliant heart surgeon since Christian Barnard, but you know less about people than...," he seemed to be stretching for a comparison, then to be surprised by the one he came up with: "than James Bonar Auldfield."

"What am I missing?" Carras said.

"Only the obvious," Vance said. "There is no third world volunteer getting paid to give up his heart. The donor is Terry Flynnt."

Carras stared at the old man. He knew his jaw had dropped open but it was a moment before he thought to close his mouth.

"That's right," Flynnt said. "I'm the only compatible donor. You're going to take my heart and put it in my son's chest. I let my father die; I will not let my son go. He's going to live, no matter what."

"No," Carras said. The refusal came without thought and he knew it came from deep within him. He didn't want to think about what the billionaire had said; if Flynnt was telling the truth, then things were not what Carras had thought they were. Flynnt was not what Carras had thought him to be.

"No," he said again. "I don't believe you. This is just another part of your game. You have to win this because you have to win everything. It's not about

Philip. If he lives, he'll take your empire apart, sell it to the highest bidder and build hospitals for kids like the ones I delivered in Haiti."

"You stupid man," Flynnt said. Do you think I give a damn what my boy does with all this," he waved at the walls around them, and Carras saw that the man's hand shook, "after I'm dead? This is nothing. The boy is everything."

"I don't believe you. With you it's always about the use of power—your power, your use."

"I think you're wrong, Ath," Charlie Vance said.

"Stay out of this, Charlie," Carras said.

"Yes, stay out of it, doctor," Flynnt said. "There's no room for a moral philosopher in this fight. For your friend, this is not about right and wrong. It's about who's going to win. And it has to be him."

"It is very much about right and wrong," Carras said.

"Only because it's about what's wrong with you," said Flynnt. "And that's a wrong so deeply set you may never want to root it out."

"What are you talking about?" Carras said. He could feel the anger rising in him but behind the hot emotion was something cold—a fear. He realized he was afraid of this man, not of what he might do but of what he might say.

"You think I just checked out your resume, doctor?" Flynnt said. He shook his head, "Nuh uh. I had people take a deep look at you. You know what they found? You like to win. Hell, you *have* to win."

There was something peculiar going on inside Athan Carras. A part of him had mentally stepped aside and was watching this confrontation as if he were a fourth person in the little room. He knew that something was going to happen here, any minute now, right here, and he knew that the thought of what might be coming was scaring the hell out of Athan Carras, scaring him into a hot, red anger that buried the fear like lava flowing over an unmarked grave. He heard himself say, "That's not true. When the oversight committee ruled against me, I submitted."

Flynnt snorted. "I read the transcript of the hearing, doctor. You took the high ground by agreeing with them. You could have brought in a lawyer to argue technicalities. But, no, that would have been victory on points. You had to have a knock-out or nothing. So you wrapped yourself in an ethical cloak and played the willing martyr. Remember, doctor, I had a Catholic school education—I recognize the type."

"You're wrong." But the dispassionate voice in Carras's head said, "Is he?"

"I'm not wrong," said Flynnt. "I also know a raging egotist when I see one. Hell, I've been one myself, all my life. Comes with being brilliant at something useful. That business on the bicycles, sure I did that because I couldn't resist taking some air out of the puffed-up balloon of your self-esteem. But I also wanted to show you that my heart was in good shape."

"You didn't mention it," Carras said.

"I realized I'd made a dumb mistake. I should have kissed your ass the way Hilary Cartiere did. She had you ready to dump your career and run off to paradise with her."

"No." Not much conviction there, said the commentator in Carras's head.

"Sure she did. But it was too late for me to change tack. So I gave you a couple of days to see if you'd come around, then I set out to do it the hard way. I had no time to lose. I had to break you down."

"But you didn't." This time the inner commentator noted the cockiness and again heard the fear it masked.

"No, I didn't," said Flynnt. "I'll give you this, doctor, your arrogance is not unfounded. You're a hell of a surgeon and my father would have called you a hell of a man. If you ever learn to bend, you might be an exceptional human being. As it is, you're at best a deeply flawed work in progress and I don't have time—my son doesn't have time—to wait for you to find your humanity."

There was a phone on the table next to the bunk. It rang and Flynnt answered it, then he said, "We're out past the three-mile limit. The legalities no longer apply. Can you really say it's wrong for me to give my life for my son?"

"I still won't do it," Carras said.

"I would, if I had the skill," Charlie Vance said. "Please, Ath. Reconsider."

But Carras shook his head. The dispassionate observer within him saw that the refusal was based not on anger but on the fear that had been growing behind the masking rage. Terry Flynnt had taken him to a place he'd never wanted to go, up onto a high point from which he could see the whole sweep of his life. And what a bleak vision it was: a man who had reduced his life to nothing but his work, a life without wife or child, with but a single friend, where every peer was a rival and no one could be allowed to surpass the lonely, driven figure on the heights. Driven, yes, but not by the needs of those he healed and saved, but by his own need to be the healer and savior—to be the one who made all the difference, the one who left behind the legacy of innovative surgical procedures that would save lives long after he was gone.

It was not a vision Athan Carras wanted to embrace. The prospect of having to admit that he had thrown away so many years, thrown away the woman and child who had loved him, terrified him. To say yes to Flynnt's revelation was to admit that he had been a fool, a prideful buffoon collecting his wall full of plaques and going home to an empty apartment that was only scarcely less empty when he was in it. He had to say no to that image of himself, to Flynnt, to Charlie Vance if his friend took the other man's side. "No," he said.

"I beg you," Flynnt said. "Not for me. For my son."

"Ath, for God's sake," Vance said. "Reconsider."

But the fear was too much. Carras turned away from the vision, his throat dry, and said, "No."

Flynnt said, "I had hoped it wouldn't come to this." He got up and squeezed past the two doctors, went to the door of the small cabin and opened it. "Your damnable pride won't let you bend even when a man begs you for his son's life. Then let us see how high a price you're willing to put on that pride."

He opened the door. In the hallway stood a young man, his hands and arms pinioned behind him, his face ashen with strain, a face Carras recognized from ten years of Christmas and birthday photographs. Isaac Dumoulin, his features impassive, held a pistol to the young man's temple.

"All right," Flynnt said. "Now it's as simple as it can be. If my son dies, so does yours."

Costas Carras looked at his father, his brown eyes ringed by an expanse of white, his limbs trembling in their bonds.

"Dad?" he said.

"Costas," Carras said. He took a step toward his son but Isaac shook his head and cocked the pistol.

"Choose," Flynnt said.

Chapter 15

I have found no evidence of a crime either being committed or planned on Bahamian territory, sir." The RBPF superintendent was speaking into a cell phone. His dark face turned toward Leonard Maigrot and took on a speculative expression as he paused to listen, then he said, "No, I am not sure that a charge of wasting police time is indicated against the complainant. At least, not yet."

A trickle of sweat tickled its way down Maigrot's back. He looked away from the policeman and found himself eye to eye with Victor Whitehall. His new employer was clearly not pleased.

"Mr. Flynnt's yacht is in international waters," the superintendent was saying. "Do you wish me to pursue it?"

The policeman folded the phone and put it away in the side pocket of his blindingly white uniform tunic. "I'm sorry, sir," he said to Whitehall, "but I am ordered to return to Nassau."

"Not until I have spoken to your Minister of State Security," Whitehall said.

"That was the Minister I was just speaking to, sir," said the policeman. "I think you will find he is now in conference and cannot be reached." He

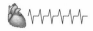

beckoned to his men and motioned them to get back into the helicopter that sat on the lawn in front of Terry Flynnt's residence complex then turned to Whitehall. "I'm concerned that you might be trespassing, sir."

"We're leaving," the old man said. He got back into the Range Rover they had found at the airport. They had driven it at breakneck speed to the wharf on the west side of the island only to see the yacht well out at sea. "We'll leave the vehicle down by the beach."

The superintendent looked to the man in sunglasses who had identified himself as the one in charge of the island in its owner's absence. The security man nodded. The policeman saluted no one in particular and permitted himself a very small smile as he climbed into the helicopter.

"What do we do now?" Maigrot asked as they went down the hill. There were six of them in the car, including the lawyer Pennock and two men that Larkin had brought along. The three black clad operatives made Maigrot nervous. They had bristle-short haircuts and muscular arms tattooed with daggers and lightning bolts. He thought that they looked at him the way well trained attack dogs might regard someone they could be at any moment commanded to savage.

"How well do you know the yacht?" Larkin said.

"Pretty well," Maigrot said.

"How many crew?"

"If there are lots of guests on board, a dozen or more stewards and cooks and so on. But when it's just Flynnt, there's often only the captain, one mate and maybe a steward."

Whitehall said, "On a ship that big?"

"All the systems are computerized," Maigrot said. "Two men can run the whole thing from the bridge."

"If they're operating on Philip Flynnt, where is that likely to take place?" Larkin said.

Maigrot didn't want to say he didn't know. He'd been in most places on the ship at one time or another and hadn't seen anything like an operating room. But there was a locked door that led down from the big lounge at the back of the boat. He told the ex-SBS man about it.

"That'll be it," Larkin said. "Where's the ship's generator?"

"There are two of them," Maigrot said. "One on either side of the engine room, about the middle of the ship."

One of the associates, a man whose face was all sharp planes, said, "The operating room might have an independent generator, just in case."

"What about it?" Larkin asked Maigrot. "Is Flynnt the just-in-case type?"

"Isaac Dumoulin is," Maigrot said.

"What about sea cocks?" said Larkin's other man, a pale eyed man with a downturned black mustache. "If the operating room's well below decks..."

"Well?" said Larkin, looking at Maigrot.

Maigrot knew he shouldn't have said what came next but Larkin and Whitehall made him so nervous that he was losing his grip on his tongue. "What are you going to do?"

"What he's paid for," said Whitehall. "And so will you. Now answer the question."

"There are two sea cocks in the engine room, too," Maigrot said. He had seen the big valves that could be opened to let in sea water to cool the engines and flush out the bilges.

"What's the easiest way there?" Larkin said.

"There's a companionway that leads down directly from the bridge."

Whitehall grunted. Larkin nodded and said, "Well, that's that then."

The trickle of sweat on Maigrot's back became a flood. He was afraid to think about just what kind of dog he had landed on this time.

• • •

The photographs of Costas hadn't done him justice, Carras thought, knowing even as the thought came to his mind that it was an aberrant observation for a father who was seeing his son for the first time in ten years—and seeing him with a cocked gun to his head when the man holding the gun looked fully able to pull the trigger. But the impression that struck Carras first and most sharply was of the intensity in the young man's face—there was strength there, and intelligence—even brilliance—and an energy that seemed to emanate from the dark eyes.

"Dad?" Costas said again, "what's happening? Who are these guys? They said you'd sent them then the next thing I know I'm on a jet and this one has a gun."

"It's all right," Carras said. "Everything's going to be fine." He felt a great need to reassure his son, as if Costas was a little boy who'd come out of his room at night still trailing the threads of a nightmare. But it was Carras who felt he was wrapped in a bad dream, his own voice sounding distant and faint in his ears.

Flynnt wasn't going to give him the leisure to work through his shock and confusion. "I said, 'Choose,' doctor," the billionaire said.

"You can't do this," Carras said.

"You can't avoid it any further," Flynnt said. "Time to see what price you put on your pride." He motioned with his head to Isaac and said, "We should do this out on deck." To Carras he said, "Come on."

"Wait," Charlie Vance said. "You can see he's in shock. Let me talk to him."

Flynnt considered. "We'll be upstairs. You've got five minutes."

"Sit down, Ath," Vance said when they were alone. He led Carras to the bed and got him seated. The cabin had a tiny washroom and Vance brought Carras a glass of water.

"What do I do, Charlie?"

"What can you do? He's got your son."

Carras stared at the wall.

"Listen, Ath," Vance said, "whatever this has been about, it's over now. We had the philosophical debate back in Miami. Now it doesn't matter whether Flynnt has the moral right to die to save his son. You do see that?"

Carras said nothing.

"Come on, Ath. We're past moral questions," Vance said. "This is about whether your son lives or dies. And if you have a problem making up your mind, then it looks to me as if Flynnt's reading of you is valid. So, tell me, is he right?"

Carras groaned.

"This can't be about you anymore," Vance said. "This has to be about Costas. Will you let him die to save your pride?" He put his hand on the surgeon's arm to urge him up.

Carras stood. His knees had gone soft, his legs felt only remotely connected to his body. There seemed to be a great silence in the air around him. The quiet commentator in his head watched as his body seemed to move in slow motion.

When they went up the stairs and through the lounge it was like a dream, like a scene from a movie. That's how you want it to be, the detached observer in his head commented. You don't want to have to deal with it.

Flynnt and Isaac had his son out on the wide rear deck. They had turned Costas so that his back was to the aft rail, below him the roiling wake of the yacht's twin screws. Flynnt stood to one side of the bound young man, Isaac to the other. The pistol hung loosely, almost negligently, in the security chief's hand.

As he approached them Carras felt as if he was sinking into an even deeper sense of unreality. His feet did not seem to touch the carpet or the rough gray paint that covered the aft deck. He was walking steadily forward but not feeling his heels strike the surfaces beneath them. He was vaguely aware of Charlie Vance beside him, but at the same time he had a sense of being completely alone.

"So," said Flynnt, "you won't take my life to save my son's. You want me to believe—you probably want to believe it yourself—that it's moral purity talking. Well, I say it's nothing but vanity, the old sin, and I know what I'm talking about. I've been like you my whole life, never gave an inch, never quit till I'd won. Until the day when I had to look into my only son's face and see him dying. That's the point where all the pride in the world can't save you, and that's the point I've brought you to. This is where the bullshit walks. You're all bluff, Carras, and I call."

Deal with it, said the voice in Carras's head. *Will you throw away your son once again—once and for all—rather than face up to what kind of man you are?*

He came to where they waited by the rail. Now he was right there, right at the decision point. Flynnt's eyes were boring into him, daring him. Isaac's gaze was as impassive as ever. The expression on Costas's face was of deepening confusion.

"What do they want, dad?" he said. "Whatever it is, just give it to them."

Carras wanted to say, *All right, you win, I'll do what you want.* He could hear the words in his mind, could almost see them as if they were wavering letters projected against a screen inside his head. But his mouth didn't open, and the words didn't come. *What's wrong with you?* the voice in his head shouted at him.

Then Isaac looked to his side, over the wake and beyond to where Forlorn Island was a dark smudge on the horizon. It was only a moment's glance, as if some motion had caught his eye, but in that moment Carras moved with a speed and precision that surprised even him.

The thumb and first two fingers of his right hand went to Isaac's wrist, unerringly finding the pressure point that controlled the man's grip on the pistol. Carras squeezed and the security chief's hand reflexively opened. The gun fell, but Carras caught it and stepped back, the muzzle pointed at Terry Flynnt's chest.

"Step away from my son," Carras said, and now his voice sounded real to him again. "Costas, come here. Get behind me."

The young man did as he was bidden. Flynnt had cocked his head to one side and was regarding Carras with a considering gaze. "So," he said, "the shock wore off pretty fast, didn't it?"

"Turn this ship around and take us back to the island," Carras said.

"Or what?" Flynnt said in a tone that indicated only mild interest whatever Carras might answer.

"Or I'll shoot you."

Flynnt and Isaac looked at each other as if Carras had just confirmed their expectations. "You'll just have to shoot me, then," said Flynnt. "We're not going anywhere but down to that operating room to save my son's life."

"I mean what I say," said Carras. "I've had enough of your games."

"No, you haven't," said the billionaire. "Fact is, at this moment you're loving this game, because now you think you're winning it."

"Turn the ship around."

"I will not. And now I'm going to come and take that gun off you, so if you've got what it takes to shoot a man now would be the time."

He stepped forward and put his hand out.

"Stop!" Carras said.

"No," said Flynnt. "Here I come."

He took another step and Carras fired.

• • •

"There are people on the aft deck," said Larkin. "I can see Flynnt and Isaac with two or three others." He lowered the binoculars and turned to Maigrot. "What does the heart doctor look like?"

Maigrot described Carras.

"He's definitely one of them," said Larkin.

"That means they haven't done the operation yet," said Victor Whitehall. "Let's keep our distance. We catch them doing something illegal on company property, we got 'em." He looked to Arthur Pennock. The lawyer nodded.

"Or maybe we just wait until they're too far out on a limb," said Larkin. He eased off the throttle and the boat's bow settled deeper into the water.

"That could work, too," said Whitehall.

• • •

A small dark hole appeared in the front of Terry Flynnt's shirt. Wisps of smoke rose from the hole's circumference, then Carras was astonished to see the hole detach itself and fall to the deck. The billionaire, unharmed, took another step toward the surgeon and took the pistol from his hands.

"Blanks," he said, rubbing one hand on the spot where the "shot" had hit.

Now the object on the deck resolved into a fragment of charred cloth. It was still smoldering and sending up tiny tendrils of gray smoke.

"So you won't take a life, no matter what?" Flynnt said.

Carras said nothing. It had become a dream again.

Flynnt rubbed the spot on his shirt again. "Did you notice that you shot me right through the heart?" he said. "If the gun had been loaded, you'd have killed both me and Philip with one shot. So you can ruin my heart with a bullet, but you won't save it with a scalpel?"

Costas spoke up. "Is this some kind of game? What the hell is going on? Dad?"

But Carras couldn't speak.

"Your father's looking for a way to avoid seeing himself for what he is," Flynnt said. "He's spent a lifetime pretending to everybody—including himself—that he's a noble servant of his profession, instead of just another puffed up egotist. The whole overblown facade just fell in on him."

Charlie Vance said, "Ath, you're my best friend and I love you, but why can't you see that he's right? You didn't have to shoot him. You could have backed away. You shot him because you wanted to beat him. This had nothing to do with right and wrong. It was about winning. Face it and let's move on."

The remote observer continued to exist inside Athan Carras only long enough to sense the tremor building in him, a tremor that became a rumble from somewhere deep, way down in the lowest levels where the blackest pains are buried. Then the long years of repressed emotion broke loose and flooded his being. First his hands shook, then the trembling went up his arms and threw his shoulders into spasms. His knees bent and tears spurted from his eyes.

Carras put his arms around his son and said, "Oh, God, oh dear God, Costas. I'm so sorry. I should never have let you go. I was wrong. I put myself first. I should never have done that. It should have been you. You deserved a father. A better father."

Costas, his arms still bound behind him, said, "What the hell is going on? Jesus, Dad, don't cry. It'll be all right."

Carras turned to Flynnt. "Cut him loose," he said. "I'll do the operation."

"Thank God," said Flynnt and it seemed that some of the strength went out of the old man' legs. He gestured to Isaac to unbind Costas and when Carras looked he saw for the first time an emotion cross the chief of security's face.

"Thank you," Isaac said.

• • •

"They're going in," said Larkin.

"Give them time to get started," said Whitehall. "Then we'll see."

"What are you going to do?" Maigrot asked.

"Prevent a crime from occurring on the property of a corporation in which I am a major shareholder. Isn't that right, Arthur?" said Whitehall.

Pennock nodded. "I'm not versed in the law of the sea, but I would say it's a defensible position, Victor."

"Even if I'm required to use reasonable force?"

"Especially in response to force that might threaten life or limb," the lawyer said.

"There you go," Whitehall said, his small dark eyes glinting. "We're on the side of the angels."

• • •

"We're shorthanded," Carras said as they came down the companionway to the deck where the operating room was.

"I did a year's residency in anesthesiology," Vance said, "before I woke up to the attractions of philosophy."

"Okay," said Carras. "You can pass the gas while Gupta looks after the heart-lung machine. His wife can handle the tools, but I'll still need someone

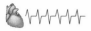

to hold the pieces while I sew them together." He looked at Costas. "Well, son, you want to see how it's done?"

Costas was rubbing his wrists and forearms where the ropes had marked them. "Sure," he said. "How can I help?"

"We'll have plenty time to talk about it after," Carras said. "For now just let me say that I've spent most of my life—and all of yours—being a fool. Today, I finally came to my senses and I'm going to do whatever I can to make it up to you. And to your mother, if she'll let me."

"I hated you," Costas said, "all those years. Because you didn't care about us. Mom always said you didn't know any better."

Carras put his hand on his son's shoulder. "That's no excuse. I should have known better. I do now. Come on, I'll show you how to scrub up."

For Carras, it was peculiar to be standing at a scrub room sink, going through all the familiar motions for the umpteenth thousandth time, but feeling as if everything was new. He was helium-light inside. It was as if he had been carrying a weight in his belly for so many years that it had become normal to be pulled down heavily toward the earth, and now the burden was plucked away and he walked with a dancer's lightness. He was as giddy as Scrooge on Christmas morning.

"You all right, Ath?" Vance said.

"Never better, Charlie."

They showed Costas how to get into the green sterile scrubs and how to wash his hands and arms thoroughly to the elbows then put on the latex gloves, flexing his fingers to get a good fit.

Dr. Gupta shouldered open the door from the OR and put his head through the gap to say that Philip Flynnt was prepped and ready, his vital signs as stable as someone in his condition could be.

"Thank you, doctor," Carras said. "We'll be right with you."

Terry Flynnt had removed his clothes except for his underwear. His body was lean and hard as an athlete's, abs and quads and lats standing out in sharp relief.

"Jesus," Costas said. "I know guys my age would kill for a body like that." Then he turned red. "Oh, God, I shouldn't have said that."

"Don't worry about it, lad," Flynnt said. "I wanted to give my son the best heart I could make for him."

Mrs. Gupta opened the OR door. "We are ready for you, sir," she said to Flynnt.

"I'll be right there," he said.

Isaac Dumoulin was standing against the door that led to the rest of the ship. Again Carras saw emotion on the normally impassive face. Flynnt turned and put his hand out to his chief of security, but Isaac reached beyond it and took his employer into his arms.

"Look after the boy," Flynnt said.

"I will," said Isaac, and there was a break in his voice.

Flynnt gently pulled himself away. His eyes were liquid. "God bless," he said and went into the operating room.

Carras said, "If you want, you can come in."

"No," Isaac said.

Carras had seen many a patient's loved ones react to the words they dreaded hearing from a surgeon—I'm sorry—but he had never seen a face more stricken than that of Isaac Dumoulin. "It will be quick and painless," Carras said.

"I'll be all right out here," Isaac said.

"Okay," Carras said and motioned for Costas to go before him into the OR. Charlie Vance had already gone ahead. The surgeon noted that his son elbowed the door open rather than touch it with his sterile gloves.

"Saw that on TV," the young man said.

"It'll be different in real life," his father said. "We won't stop every twenty minutes for commercials." The operating room was state of the art. Carras had operated and taught in ORs all over the world and this sterile, gleaming space had everything he needed—plus two things he didn't. His eyes flicked over the two atomic hearts in their cabinet. Then he put them out of his mind and focused on the procedure he was about to perform.

Terry Flynnt was on table two and Mrs. Gupta was arranging drapes to cover him except for a space on his chest, which she painted with a red-brown antiseptic solution.

"We're going to get Philip connected to the heart-lung machine," Carras said. "That'll take a few minutes. Then we take out the bad heart. Then it will be time for... for you."

"All right," Flynnt said.

"We can put you under any time."

The billionaire nodded. "I'll wait. I want to think about a few things. Remember a few things."

"Of course," said Carras. He turned to take his position to the left of the patient on table one.

"Doctor," Terry Flynnt said.

Carras turned back. "Yes?"

"My offer—the research institute, the budget, everything—it's still yours."

Carras made a little sound in his throat and shook his head. "No, thanks," he said. "I've spent all the time I intend to up on a mountain top. There are some valleys that I'm long past getting around to exploring."

"Well, then, you have my thanks," said Flynnt. "My heartfelt thanks." He laughed and for once it wasn't a humorless bark.

Carras turned back to table one, swept his eyes over the monitors. The patient's blood pressure was not good and the respiration was no better, but it was as good as it was going to get before they went in. Carras looked to Charlie Vance and Dr. Gupta. "Ready?" he said.

"Quite ready, doctor," said the Indian.

"Blaze away," said Vance.

Carras looked across the table at his son. "If you feel ill, turn your head."

"I think I'll be okay," Costas said. "I'm your son."

Carras blinked. *Focus,* he reminded himself. "Yes," he said then turned to Mrs. Gupta. "Scalpel, please."

• • •

"There's a pulled up gangway on her starboard side," Larkin said. "Got to be the easiest way aboard."

Whitehall looked at his watch. "Do it," he said.

Larkin pushed the throttle forward and the fast boat lifted its bow out of the water. The wind of their passage swept over Leonard Maigrot seated in the stern and the spray dampened his hair and clothing. The tropical sun had climbed to the top of the sky but he was chilled.

Larkin's two men opened a compartment in the side of the boat and brought out dark, bulky objects wrapped in opaque plastic. They unwrapped them to reveal the squared off utilitarian shapes of three machine pistols . The men then took long magazines out of the plastic wrap and tapped them against the deck before thrusting them into the weapons. They snapped back bolts and adjusted some kind of switch on the sides of the guns then sat with the killing machines resting on their thighs as calmly as if they were commuters on a morning train with briefcases on their knees.

Larkin brought the boat bouncing into the yacht's wake and moved it up toward the starboard side.

"Won't they see us on radar?" Maigrot said.

"The boat is coated in a radar absorbing paint," said Larkin's man, the one with the mustache.

"You want an irony, the paint's manufactured by Flynnt," said the one with the face made of sharp angles.

Maigrot didn't want an irony. He wanted to be away from here. He knew that some of the decisions he had influenced in his career must have come down at some far removal to men like these making jokes as they prepared to use their guns. But this time the removal was nil. Bullets might be about to fly toward vulnerable flesh, piercing and tearing, and although Leonard Maigrot could contemplate such things happening to anonymous others far away from his comfortable corner office, he didn't think he could bear to be where the torn flesh might turn out to be his own.

"Seasick?" said Planed Face, with no trace of concern.

"A little."

"We have a cure," said Mustache. He pointed the machine pistol at Maigrot and made his eyebrows dance.

Maigrot felt his breakfast coming up and turned to spew over the stern of the boat. Between spasms, he could hear the men laughing.

"Stand to," said Larkin. "We're there."

Maigrot turned, wiping the bitterness from his lips. They were coming up fast under the starboard stern of the big yacht, bouncing in the wake, then they shot over and past the rolling curl of water and came up hard against the ship's side.

Maigrot looked up. The gangway was parallel with the lower deck of the yacht, a long thin rectangle of metal framing painted white and wooden steps coated in sandpapery gray deck paint. It seemed very far above them.

Mustache stood up, the machine gun slung from his neck by a strap and a rope that ended in a rubber covered grapnel in his hands. He balanced himself, legs spread against the boat's bumps and surges, then swung the rope up to the gangway. The grapnel caught in the staircase's railing and both Mustache and Planed Face hauled the gangway down until its lowest step was only a foot above the boat's gunwale. Larkin eased the small craft off a foot or two, lest the turbulence smash them against the metal frame.

Mustache stood on the gunwale and stepped across the roiling sea onto the gangway. His companion followed briskly. "Now you," Larkin said to Maigrot.

He didn't want to do it. This was not the way he preferred to do business. But he had no doubt that a refusal now—even a show of reluctance—would result in his termination, and not just from Victor Whitehall's payroll.

He took a ragged breath and jumped, landing poorly and having to clutch at Larkin's two men for fear of falling into the water. Mustache grunted in disgust and thrust Maigrot up the stairs.

"You first," he said. "They know you."

Shivering from more than the damp chill, Maigrot climbed the steps.

• • •

Carras opened up Philip Flynnt's mediastinum and saw what he expected to see. The heart was severely weakened and enlarged.

Carras looked up across the table at his son. "You all right?" he said.

Costas's eyes met his. "I had a little twinge when you made the cut, but I'm okay now," he said. "It's just like circuitry. I can see how it all connects, even though I don't know the names of the parts."

"Maybe you'd make a good surgeon," Carras said.

The boy shook his head. "I think I prefer silicon."

Not long before, Carras thought, he would probably have been disappointed to hear his son say what he had just said. Now it was okay. He didn't need the vote of confidence that came from having a son following in his footsteps. It was enough just to have a son, and the kind of son who already knew what he was going to do with his life and would do it brilliantly.

He became aware of another change: His power of concentration was the same as before, yet he felt as if his being had been enlarged. He could be tightly focused on the two square feet of flesh in front of him and at the same time feel as if he somehow encompassed all the people in the room, held them in his regard even as the front part of his mind carefully managed the intricate details of open heart surgery.

It was as if he had spent so much his life living in a single room of a big house that he had forgotten—had denied—that other rooms even existed. Now suddenly the doors were open, the walls whisked away, and he was conscious of being much more than he had ever been. More than that, he knew that the one room he had thought so much of was of little account compared to the whole of the great mansion he had so long ignored.

• • •

The captain and the mate turned when the inner door to the bridge opened. The captain, a small silver haired man, said, "Mr. Maigrot, I didn't know you were aboard," and then froze as Larkin and his two men stepped inside and pointed their weapons.

"Away from the controls," said the ex-SBS man and waved the two sailors away from the panel of telltale lights and switches. "Hands behind your heads."

"What's going on?" the captain wanted to know.

Victor Whitehall and Arthur Pennock came in. At Whitehall's nod, the lawyer said, "I am Arthur Pennock, a director of the company that owns this yacht. I have reason to believe that Terry and Philip Flynnt are using it to commit a serious crime—in fact, murder—and I have authorized these men to seize control so that we may prevent the crime."

The captain wasn't fazed. "I want to talk to Mr. Flynnt," he said.

Larkin pointed his gun. "You'll talk to nobody but me," he said. "Is there any other crew aboard, stewards, engine room ratings?"

The captain looked as if he didn't want to answer, but Pennock said, "You could be charged as an accessory if you don't cooperate."

"I work for Mr. Flynnt," said the captain.

"Flynnt is finished," said Whitehall. "You work for us now. And if you don't do as you're told not only will I have these gentlemen beat you thoroughly but I will see to it that you'll lose your pension and you'll never take the wheel of anything bigger than a tugboat."

The silver haired man swallowed. He didn't like it but he gestured with his head to the mate and said, "Mick and I are the only crew aboard We were only going out a few miles then back before nightfall."

Larkin produced two pairs of handcuffs from a pouch on his belt. A minute later, the captain and mate were handcuffed to each other as well as to a chair bolted to the floor in a small cabin just aft of the bridge that was reserved for the senior officer.

"Right," said Larkin, when they were back on the bridge with the cabin door closed, "here's how we do it." He told the one with the mustache to go down the companionway to the engine room and find the sea cocks: large pipes that were used to let in sea water to flush the bilges but which, if left open, would soon fill the hull with water and sink the ship.

"We'll let her settle deep enough to kill the power to the operating room. We'll close off the door, bottle them up."

"But they might already have started the operation," Maigrot said.

"Then we would be unfortunately too late to prevent the crime," said Whitehall.

"But if we cut the power to those machines they use, Philip Flynnt might..."

"Criminals always run that kind of risk," Whitehall said. "We can't be held responsible," he looked at Pennock, "Can we?"

The lawyer shook his head.

Whitehall said to Larkin, "Get to it. Pennock and I will contact the other Flynnt Group directors and convene an emergency meeting of the board by conference call."

"What about him?" Larkin indicated Maigrot.

"Our new friend has done his part," Whitehall said, and Maigrot saw his employer weighing up the question of whether or not he could be of any more use. He let out a breath he didn't know he had been holding when Whitehall said, "Perhaps he could take the minutes of the emergency meeting."

Larkin shrugged and said to his men, "Let's go."

Maigrot was left with Whitehall and the lawyer. Pennock produced a satellite phone from a pocket and began entering numbers. Whitehall walked up and down the bridge with his hands behind his back inspecting its fittings.

"Is there anything I can do for you, sir?" Maigrot said.

"That would certainly be the question we'll need to answer, wouldn't it?" said Whitehall.

Definitely the wrong dog, thought Maigrot. *This one's picky about his fleas.* He wondered if Whitehall would be murderously picky.

Chapter 16

saac Dumoulin stood in the scrub room between the OR and the corridor that was the only connection to the rest of the ship. Bright light flooded through the round windows in the door leading to the room where Terry Flynnt was giving up his life for his son.

Isaac wanted to be in that room, knew he had a right to be there when the old man died. But his role was to defend the Flynnt family, to be the faithful guardian at the gates and now he stood as he had for thirty years, between the Flynnts and whatever might come at them.

The odds were that there was no threat right at this moment. The Bahamian police had landed on the island, looking for evidence of an illegal medical procedure, but they had gone. The RBPF might have tried to order them back to port but Flynnt had told the captain to maintain radio silence. By now they were well into international waters and should be safe from interference while the old man's will was carried out.

But who had sent the RBPF after them? Isaac picked up a surgical mask from a shelf and covered his mouth. He crossed to the door into the operating room and opened it enough to put his head through. He focused his eyes on the surgeon and deliberately did not look at what was on the table or the thing in the dish that the man was probing with a gloved hand.

"Doctor Carras?"

The surgeon looked up. "What?"

"Did you send the Bahamian police to the island?" Isaac said.

"It never occurred to me."

Isaac nodded and backed out of the door. He'd doubted that the doctor would have had the pull necessary to sic the RBPF on Flynnt. It had to be Whitehall. The question was: was Victor Whitehall the kind of man who would let the outcome of a major corporate takeover hang on a decision by some Bahamian policeman?

Isaac didn't think so. There would be a Plan B and it would be happening now. There was an intercom mounted on the wall. He pushed the buttons that opened a circuit to the bridge and said, "Captain, please call Frankl and find out what's been happening ashore."

There was no reply.

"Captain," Isaac said again. "Did you hear me?"

There was a long pause, then the captain's voice came back. "Sorry, Isaac. Little busy here. I'll call him right away."

"Thank you," Isaac said. "Anything on the radar, anything nearby?"

"Nothing special, Isaac. There's a tanker about twenty miles south of us."

"Thank you," Isaac said again. He cut the connection. Then he locked the door between the scrub room and the corridor and started to think. Hard.

• • •

In the engine room, Larkin's man spun the great wheel that opened the valve to the second sea cock. He could hear nothing over the thrumming of the giant twin diesels, but when he put his hand on the pipe below the valve he could feel the vibration caused by the rush of seawater that was now flooding the bilges in the space beneath his feet.

He looked at his watch. Larkin had said to give him and the other man five minutes to get into position. He waited until the counter on the timepiece clicked off the last second, then he shut off the diesels and threw the switches that turned off the generators. The engine room fell into silence and a darkness broken only by a bright battery powered lamp that automatically turned itself on to illuminate the stairs of the companionway. The man used the butt of his machine pistol to break the lamp's glass faceplate and the bulb behind it. The faintest glow of blue emergency lighting descended into the engine room from the door to the bridge above him.

Larkin had examined the yacht's schematics on the bridge. By the time the water rising from the bilges reached the engine room the separate generator that powered the lights and equipment in the OR would be drowned. Philip Flynnt's operation would stop, probably at an irreversible point in the procedure, which was the goal of the mission. The rest would be mopping up, Larkin had said.

• • •

Larkin and the planed-face man eased down the stairway and reached the door that opened on the corridor that led to the operating room. The plan was simple: when the main generators went out, Isaac Dumoulin and Terry Flynnt would come out of the operating room to see what had happened. They would be backlit by the lights of the OR and he and his man would shoot them. Then they would go into the OR and shoot everybody else.

Whitehall hadn't ordered it done that way, Larkin knew. Maybe the fat man thought his wealth and power could keep a lid on whatever happened here, that those who survived would be cowed into keeping quiet. Or maybe he didn't think so and knew that hiring Larkin meant that the job would be done thoroughly.

Either way, on an operation like this, the ex-SBS man had no intention of leaving behind anybody who might tell of things that were better left untold. He would arrange a fire and sink the yacht. He and the other boarders would take one of the ship's Zodiacs and find the boat he had left drifting a few miles back. They would sink the Zodiac and that would be that.

Silently, Larkin and his man went through the door at the foot of the stairway and found the corridor empty. The metal door at the other end of the passage was closed. They checked the two small cabins and found them unoccupied. Then they squatted down at the foot of the stairs to wait.

Precisely on time, the ship's engines died and moments later the lights went out. Larkin eased back the bolt on his weapon. It made only the tiniest noise.

• • •

Terry Flynnt's heart looked strong and healthy. Despite Flynnt's age, Carras saw not a shred of coronary arteriosclerosis. But Carras ran his gloved finger around the chambers and carefully inspected the organ before saying, "It's good. Let's put it in."

While Nurse Gupta held the organ in its icy bath Carras trimmed and shaped its major structures. Then Carras gently lifted the heart and deposited it on the soaked sponge that the nurse placed next to the incision in Philip's chest.

"Hold that artery for me," Carras told Costas. The young man responded well, a firm grip and no hesitation. *Good hands,* Carras thought, then concentrated on sewing the first connecting sutures.

From there on in, the transplant was as routine as an operation performed by a scratch team, including one amateur, could manage. Father and son worked together, Costas holding the arteries and veins while Carras stitched.

"That's the left atrium attached," Carras said, adding, "You're doing a good job, Costas." A few minutes later, "And the right atrium." They sewed intently, Carras and Carras. "Now we do the pulmonary artery." He looked up, saw his son's eyes bright with interest above the mask. "Last, we attach the aorta, that's this one. It provides the heart with nutrient blood and channels the heart's output to all the body's organs."

He put in the last stitch, then said, "Hmm." Since completing the suturing, the new heart had been fibrillating, erratically and ineffectively quivering. It was still doing so.

"What is it, Dad?" Costas said.

Carras touched the quivering flesh. "The moment of truth," he said, then turned to Dr. Gupta. "Lidocaine, 250 mg, please," The powerful antiar-rhythmic should have acted almost immediately. But Flynnt's heart continued to fibrillate.

"All right, let's have the paddles. Give me 10 joules." Carras put the large, fly-swatter-like paddles around the shivering heart, then nodded to the nurse. She pressed the large red button on the defibrillator. Philippe's body arched violently from the shock, but the heart did not respond.

That's not good, Athan said to himself. His mind made rapid deductions, but to the rest of the crew in the OR he showed the placid face of the ice man. "Dr. Gupta, please raise your perfusion, pressure. Give me 80 millimeters." That would see the new heart well nourished with blood, though it meant running the heart-lung machine harder, at its "red line." Carras watched the enhanced blood flow take effect. "We'll rest the heart at this higher pressure for the next fifteen minutes," he said, "and then we'll try again."

The sweep hand on the wall-mounted clock counted off the seconds as they built, achingly slowly, into minutes. In a normal operation, Carras would have chatted with his crew. But he had nothing to say to Dr. Gupta, and far too much to say to Costas, but this was not the time and place for that conversa-tion. So they stood in silence until the heart-lung machine had had its fifteen minutes to revitalize the new heart. Then Carras took up the paddles and said, "Give me 20 this time."

Again Nurse Gupta pressed the red button, again the body arched from the shock. This time the heart stopped fibrillating, even took a few tentative normal beats, then the fibrillation began again. Carras swore silently. Could all of this be for nothing?

He fought off the doubt, let the ice man take control. "Let's repeat, this time ready to pace atrially," he said. "We'll convert again with the counter-shock, but this time I want to gently pace the upper chambers of the heart to maintain an organized heartbeat longer." Again he positioned the paddles, again came the high, arching, seizure-like, almost barbaric arching of Philip's body, and again a few tentative, irregularly timed, but effective heartbeats.

"Pace. Pace now." he said, giving Dr. Gupta the precise settings for the pacemaker. "Asynchronous, rate 120, full output."

The tentative, irregular beats gave way to a regular, precisely timed, and effective rhythm. The heart grew visibly stronger with each pulsation. Within minutes, it was almost jumping out of the chest with strength. The new heart, supplied with oxygen-rich blood from the heart-lung machine, and yet to have any load imposed on it, was restoring itself, discarding the toxic metabolites that had built up during the time when it had languished during implantation without blood flow, replenishing the energy stores of its tireless muscle cells.

The old man's heart beat in the young man's chest. Carras instructed Dr. Gupta to wean the patient off bypass. Now came another, the final, moment of truth. Now the new heart would be asked not only to beat rhythmically but also to take on the burden of actually pumping the blood to Philip's body. Carras watched as the heart-lung machine tapered off and the new heart took to its task effortlessly. Within moments, it was pumping vigorously, generating a blood flow three times any level of output that the old heart had been able to manage for years.

"Houston, we have lift-off," Carras said. He began to disconnect the heart-lung machine tubings. In a moment, he would turn his skills to closing the chest layers, a process he could have done in his sleep. He glanced at the clock. It was the middle of the night. Only now, with his patient safe, did he let the ice man fade away so that Athan Carras could think about what else was transpiring on the ship, outside the floating OR and on the upper decks.

Isaac felt the muted rumble of the ship's engines cease. A moment later, the fluorescent lights in the scrub room went out though the flood of light through the round window in the door to the OR did not diminish. Then he heard the noise from the corridor, the tiny click of metal on metal. He knew instantly what it was. And what it meant.

He put the sterile mask over his mouth again and pushed the door to the OR partly open. "Everything all right in here?" he said.

Carras looked up, but only for a moment. "Yep," he said.

"We've got a problem," Isaac said. "Some people are on the ship. They've got the bridge and they're out in the corridor with guns. They're not the police."

Carras said, "They're Victor Whitehall's people?"

The doctor was always surprising Isaac. "You know about that?"

Carras's hands were busy inside Philip Flynnt's chest. "Yeah," he said. "What are they going to do?"

"Kill us all," Isaac said, "if they can."

"What are you going to do?"

"Kill them first. If I can."

Carras looked up again. "Good luck," he said. "Anything we can do?"

"Stay here. But if the lights go out and water starts coming in, try and get the hell out."

"You think they're going to sink the ship?"

"It's how they'll get rid of the evidence," Isaac said. He thought for a moment then said, "Have you got a heavyweight scalpel?"

Carras didn't look up this time. He said, "Nurse Gupta, give him a Number 10 scalpel."

The woman didn't move. Isaac saw that she was too scared to respond.

Now the surgeon looked up. "Nurse," he said, and his tone made her jump. "Do your job."

The Indian woman took an instrument from a tray on a table and offered it handle first to Isaac. He took it and backed out of the door.

• • •

Isaac Dumoulin cut a hole in the wall of the scrub room. The yacht's surgical facility had been built as one self-contained compartment, hung from gymbals so that it would remain unmoving even if the ship was being tossed about by heavy seas. To save weight, the walls within the large metal box that housed the operating and scrub rooms as well as the two small cabins fitted out as recovery rooms were made of ordinary plasterboard over spiderweb aluminum studs. It took only moments for the scalpel to cut through the paper and plaster.

He emerged into the tiny washroom attached to the recovery room. The darkness was complete except for small blue emergency lights set into the walls just above the floor. The door into the cabin was open. Silently, Isaac crossed the small space and put his ear against the wall that separated the room from the corridor. He heard nothing. But that's where they'll be, he thought. That's where I'd be.

He drew the automatic pistol from its shoulder holster. It was not the one he'd let the doctor take from him—nicely done, that pressure point trick, he admitted—but his favorite piece, a SIG Sauer P226 with fifteen nine milli-meter Luger rounds in the clip.

Isaac transferred the pistol to his left hand and picked a spot on the wall. He began to make a peep hole with the surgical steel.

• • •

Something was bothering Leonard Maigrot. It wasn't that he had betrayed his employer or even that he was now permanently attached to a man who made sharks look tender hearted. But something had triggered a mental relay deep in Maigrot's danger-recognition circuits, the early warning system that since his fear-raddled childhood had served to tell him when pain was coming his way.

He closed his eyes and let the information come up from wherever inside his mind crouched the perpetually frightened little boy who was the real core of Maigrot's being. And, reliably, the knowledge came.

"Isaac knows we're here," he said.

Victor Whitehall stopped his pacing and turned his porcine eyes on Maigrot. "How does he know?"

"The captain, he called him Isaac," Maigrot said. "Twice. He always calls him Mr. Dumoulin."

Whitehall looked toward the closed door of the ready room where the captain and mate were again handcuffed to a post. Maigrot saw a murderous rage fill the fat man's face, then saw the emotion swiftly put down as Whitehall turned back to him. "What will he do?"

The answer was a distant roar of gunfire from aft.

Maigrot's voice sounded as if there was not enough breath in him to form the words. "He'll come here and kill us."

• • •

Isaac had waited until his eyes adjusted to the darkness before peeking through the tiny hole he had made in the plasterboard. Even so, at first all he saw was blackness. Whoever they were, they knew how to keep still. Professionals, he thought, military training, probably ex-special forces.

He put his ear to the hole and listened. It was soft, but he heard someone breathing. *Surely there'll be more than one.* He put his eye back again and waited. They didn't know they were being looked for. They would move, adjust their positions as limbs stiffened toward cramp. He waited, then waited some more, and then it came.

It was blackness against blackness, but a darker shade against a lighter, and when the man crouched against the far wall of the corridor moved, Isaac sensed it. Now he knew: if there was only one of them, he had seen where the man was. If there were two, the only safe position for the second man was on his side of the corridor, right below the hole Isaac was looking through.

The security chief transferred the SIG Sauer to his right hand and placed the palm of the left over the small hole, just in case a gleam of blue might shine through to the corridor. Then he kneeled and placed the muzzle of the pistol against the thin stuff of the wall where the second man's head would be if there was a second man.

The weapon was already cocked. Isaac pulled the trigger and emptied the magazine through the wall. Then he popped the clip, slid in a fresh load, opened the door and put the SIG Sauer out into the corridor and emptied the second clip. Only when he had a third magazine in place did he roll through the door, land on his belly and aim at the huddled shapes at the foot of the staircase to the lounge.

They weren't moving now.

• • •

In the OR the blast of gunfire was very loud, even through the two sets of doors. Carras was closing up Philip Flynnt's chest, his fingers smoothly going through the sequence of suturing. Costas was holding the edges of severed flesh together, and the young man's hands did not flinch when the thunder of violence erupted only a few feet away, although the Indian woman screamed.

"How are we doing, people?" Carras said.

"I don't think I'd book with this cruise line again," Charlie Vance said.

Dr. Gupta had put his arms around his wife and was making shushing noises as his hands patted her back. "At this moment, a little practice in New Delhi is not so unappealing," he said.

Isaac Dumoulin's masked face appeared around the edge of the door to the scrub room. "We're still in the game," he said. "But everybody stay here."

"Sure," said Carras. "We've got our hands full anyway."

He set and tied off another suture and looked at his son. Flynnt had been right: the stuff the world gave you—fame, prestige, plaques on the wall—it was nothing compared to this.

"So," he said, "silicon addict, huh?"

"Yep," said Costas.

"Well, that's all right. Maybe you could teach me about it a little."

His son smiled. "Glad to."

• • •

"Now it makes sense," Isaac said as he stepped onto the crescent shaped bridge through the door on the starboard side and saw Leonard Maigrot with Whitehall and Pennock. "You always had the smell of a Judas on you."

"You didn't give me any choice," Maigrot said. "You don't tell me what's going on, what am I supposed to do?"

"Be loyal to the man who paid you."

"Never mind him," said Victor Whitehall. "The man who's been paying you is finished. I'm taking this company. I've called an emergency meeting of the board of directors by conference call and it begins in five minutes. Five minutes after that, you'll be working for me."

"Not in this lifetime," said Isaac.

Whitehall went on as if he hadn't spoken. "The fact that you're here impresses me. I heard the gunfire. That means Larkin is no longer available. I will pay you twice whatever you were getting from Flynnt."

"Forget it," said Isaac. His eyes moved over the three men. There was something wrong here. Pennock and Maigrot were scared stiff, like they ought to be. But Whitehall was acting as if he was still running the game. He must know that this was no longer about board meetings and proxies.

The bridge was crescent shaped, not a big space, dominated by the forward windows and the bank of controls lit by their own illumination. Two battery powered emergency lamps made cones of brightness against the rear wall. The lawyer and the weasel were standing stock still in the middle of the floor. Whitehall was off to one side.

"Where's the crew?" Isaac said.

Whitehall indicated the door to the ready room. "We locked them up," he said.

"Now you can let them out."

"They're handcuffed to a post. Larkin has the key."

Isaac hefted the SIG Sauer. "Then we'll do it cowboy style." He lifted his chin toward the lawyer. "Open it," he said.

Pennock did as he was told. Through the open door Isaac saw the captain and the mate sitting on the floor, handcuffed as Whitehall had said. Their mouths were taped.

"Okay," he said, "all of you into the ready room."

"It'll be a pretty tight fit," said Whitehall.

"We'd have more room if I just shoot you right here," Isaac said.

He motioned them into the little room then crossed the width of the bridge. The door in the middle of the rear wall, the one that opened on the companionway down to the engine room was closed. Isaac flicked the button that locked it as he went by.

The fat man had been right: there wasn't much room in the little compartment off the bridge. Just a bunk, a table with one chair and a couple of lockers. Isaac crowded the three men against the far wall and told Maigrot to hand him a pillow from the bunk.

Isaac told the captain and mate to put their connected hands down on the deck. He placed the pillow over the handcuff chain and positioned the muzzle of the pistol over the links. Now the round would go into the wooden deck and the pillow would catch any flying debris.

Both crewmen were making noises behind their gags, wriggling around. "Don't worry," he said, and then he noticed that Whitehall was moving.

It wasn't any sudden motion, only that the fat man was sliding himself between Leonard Maigrot and the back wall. And now Maigrot and the lawyer looked very scared.

It all clicked in Isaac's head. They had a key to the handcuffs; they'd freed the captain to talk to him on the intercom while Larkin was waiting outside the OR. They'd lied to him because they wanted him in this little room.

Why gag the two crew? The answer came: to keep them from telling him about the man in one of the lockers behind him. The man with the gun.

Even as he was thinking it, Isaac threw himself down and to the left, seeing Whitehall grab Maigrot by the shoulders and prevent the turncoat from getting out of the line of fire of Larkin's man who was now spraying the little room with an automatic weapon.

Isaac felt the bullets stitch through his right shoulder and upper arm. They were high velocity rounds and he felt them tear flesh from his body. The pistol fell from his nerveless right hand—just like the doctor he thought—but he caught it with his left and rolled over onto his screaming wounded limb.

The gunman was coming out of the cramped locker to get a clear shot at Isaac and finish the job. The security chief had only time to see the man's slitted eyes and the dark line of his mustache before he fired three shots that obliterated the target's face in a red-white-pink spray of blood, bone and brains.

The pain was shrieking in his arm and shoulder, but Isaac rolled back onto his left side and managed to lever himself into a sitting position, the unwounded side of his back braced against the wall. He put the muzzle of the gun against the chain beneath the pillow and fired once. The links parted and the captain and mate were half free. He handed the captain the pistol. Another shot and the job was done.

"Are we sinking?" Isaac said.

The captain pulled away the tape on his mouth and said, "I think so."

"Then stop it."

"What about your wounds?"

"First things first."

"Aye, aye, Mr. Dumoulin." The captain motioned with his head to tell the mate to follow him onto the bridge.

Isaac looked around the small room. The gunman's rounds had gone high and Pennock had been dropping to the floor the moment the locker door opened. He was unhurt but he wasn't going to move again until he was sure it was all over. His face was pressed to the deck and his body was trembling.

Leonard Maigrot was in pieces. He'd taken several hits, high powered rounds that had torn up his shirt front and everything underneath. Isaac could see fragments of shattered bone where the man's chest used to be. His throat was ripped away and his jaw bone was beside him on the floor. He was very dead.

Victor Whitehall was sitting with his back against the wall, legs extended and chin slumped on his wide chest. He looked liked an overstuffed bean bag doll some kid had abandoned. Blood was leaking from wounds in his torso, but when Isaac checked them he saw that the perforations were shallow. Leonard Maigrot had been useful for once.

The fat man shuddered and took a long, gobbly breath. His eyes opened and fixed on the security chief. "Help me," he said. "I'll make it worth your while."

Isaac turned to the lawyer huddled on the deck. "You," he said. "Get your ass over here and help me up."

It hurt to stand, but he found he could walk all right. He indicated Whitehall with the pistol. "Now get him up."

Pennock squatted, put one of Whitehall's arms over his shoulder and, grunting, managed to get to his feet.

"Bring him along," Isaac said and limped as he led the way aft.

• • •

Carras was preparing to move Philip into one of the small cabins set up as intensive care units when the door to the OR opened. "I got fresh business for you," Isaac Dumoulin said.

"Jesus," Carras said, "what happened to you?" The man's right side was soaked in blood, the arm dangling uselessly.

"Not me," he said. "Out here."

In the scrub room, Pennock was gasping for breath, but only from the exertion of having lugged Victor Whitehall's mass of flesh from the bridge. The tycoon was sitting on the floor, his chest soaked in blood but his eyes locked onto the doctor.

"You're the heart surgeon?" Whitehall said.

"I'm Dr. Athan Carras."

"And you've just performed an illegal operation?"

"I transplanted Terry Flynnt's heart into his son, Philip."

The news caught Whitehall by surprise but he recovered fast. "Flynnt's dead?"

"What do you think?" Carras said.

"But Philip's out of commission for a while?"

"He'll recover soon."

Whitehall turned his head toward Pennock. "Get on the phone," he said. "Convene that emergency meeting pronto."

Pennock felt his pockets.

Isaac said, "You looking for this?" and held up the shattered remains of the lawyer's satellite phone.

Whitehall said, "I demand you provide me access to communications."

"You can demand all you want," Isaac said, "but go near a phone on this boat without Mr. Philip Flynnt gives his permission and I'll shoot you." He looked at Pennock. "Same goes for you."

"You have no right," the lawyer began, but Isaac cut him off.

"You boarded us in international waters and forced the captain to give up command at gunpoint. That makes you pirates, and I'm within my rights to shoot you dead."

"I'm a major shareholder of the company that owns this yacht and he's a director," Whitehall said. "We had every right to come aboard. Any court would uphold us."

"In that case, your deaths will have been a tragic accident," Isaac said. He turned to Carras. "Can you patch me up? I got to watch these bastards until Frankl can get out here with a crew."

"No problem," Carras said.

"You can't stop me from taking the Flynnt Group," Whitehall said. "It's just a matter of time."

"That'll be up to Philip," Isaac said. "Meantime, we wait."

• • •

By evening, Whitehall and Pennock, the former's shallow wounds treated, were confined to cabins guarded by Frankl and one of his olive clad security men. Isaac was resting in his own cabin, his wounds stitched and bandaged and a pint of blood transfused through his system. His blood type was the same as the Flynnts', enabling him to receive some of the supply that had been put aside for the operation.

Costas called his mother from the bridge. Night was coming on in the Bahamas, but it was afternoon in California. When he told her where he was, she was speechless. The last she'd seen him had been that morning. He'd been on his way to school for an early morning class. It was in one of the big anonymous Stanford parking lots that Isaac Dumoulin had approached the young man and spun him the tale about taking him to his father.

"Are you all right?" his mother said.

"Never better," Costas answered. "I'm with Dad."

"Your father's there?"

"Yep."

"How are you getting along?"

"He's pretty cool," Costas said. "We'll be home in a few days."

• • •

Early next morning, Carras made his rounds, beginning with Philip Flynnt. The Guptas had taken turns watching the patient through the night and all the data were waiting for Carras when he arrived. The figures for pulse, blood pressure, urine output, pressures in the heart and bleeding from the chest drains were all solidly in the normal range.

Philip had awakened an hour before and the Guptas had weaned him from the breathing tube. Now he was sleeping quietly, his wife seated beside the bed, holding his hand. She had come from the island with Frankl.

"He's going to be all right, isn't he?" Annabella asked. She looked dazed, as if the events of the past twenty-four hours had pushed her back a half-step from reality.

"He's going to be fine," Carras said.

"When he woke up, he wanted to know what his father had done. He thought there'd been some kind of awful black-market deal. But Dr. Gupta told me what happened and I told Philip."

"How did he take it?"

"He cried. He wished he'd known."

"But if he'd known what his father wanted to do," Carras said, "Philip would have tried to stop it."

Annabella wiped the tears that misted her eyes. She didn't look like a cover girl this morning, Carras thought. Just a woman who'd found, against all hope, that her dying man would live. "The last words they ever spoke to each other were pretty harsh. Philip wished he could take them back."

"Give it time," Carras said. "These things have a way of working themselves out."

Costas came in. "I've been looking for you," he said. "The security man says that Whitehall guy is demanding to see you."

"He can wait. I have more needful patients."

"Anything I can do?" the young man said.

"Would you mind staying here with Mr. and Mrs. Flynnt? I think she could use the company."

Annabella said, "I could."

"Sure," Costas said. "You know, you look familiar. Have I seen you somewhere before?"

"Probably," she said.

• • •

By the time Carras got to Whitehall's cabin, the fat man was furious. "I'll ruin you," he said by way of greeting.

Carras checked the man's signs and examined the wounds. The worst of them, a jagged rip where Carras had had to remove one of Leonard Maigrot's teeth from Whitehall's upper chest, was showing no sign of infection. "Well, you'll soon be completely recovered," he said. "You can get back to ruining lives at full bore."

Whitehall changed tack. "Get me out of here and I'll make it worth your while."

"It's not my say," Carras told him. "But Isaac asked me to tell you that he's set up a meeting of the Flynnt Group board for tomorrow afternoon."

"Where?"

"Here, on the yacht."

Now Whitehall smiled and Carras did not find it a pleasant sight. "Then we'll settle this once and for all," the fat man said.

"I think that's the general idea." Carras made to leave, then turned back. "It doesn't bother you that four men are dead because of you?"

"They knew the risks," Whitehall said. "If it bothers you, doctor, you're mixing with the wrong kind of people. Flynnt's killed his share."

• • •

Isaac sent the Boeing to bring the four directors down to Forlorn Island, the three fund managers from New York and the retired two-star general from Washington. A motor launch brought them to where the yacht pursued a figure eight course in the wide stretch of ocean between Florida and the Bahamas.

The yacht's spacious boardroom took up the rear half of the topmost deck, a wide windowed space dominated by a long rectangular table of blond wood with darker inlay, set around with plush armchairs that moved easily across the deep carpet on ghost-silent castors. Philip Flynnt was not well enough to occupy one of the chairs; instead, his bed had been brought up by the elevator that opened on the forward end of the big room. Carras and Costas maneuvered the bed to the head of the table, and it was there that Whitehall and Pennock found the young man when Isaac brought them up along with the other directors. The security chief's arm was in a sling but if he was in any pain it didn't show.

"Why is Philip Flynnt in the chairman's position?" was the first thing Whitehall said when they were seated.

"Because I am chairing the meeting," Philip said, his voice soft but firm. "For that matter, who are you to ask questions, Whitehall? You're not a director of this company."

"Not yet," Whitehall said. He nudged Pennock, who said, "Mr Whitehall is a significant shareholder..."

"Twenty-one percent," Whitehall said, and the folds of skin around his sharp little eyes moved to emphasize his satisfaction.

"My father has always been the chairman of this company," Philip began. "He founded it."

"He's dead," Pennock said, prompted by another nudge from his owner.

"I am his heir and will inherit his shares," Philip told the lawyer.

"But until the will goes through probate, you don't control them. So you can't vote them today."

Isaac Dumoulin had been standing beside the elevator door. Now he took a seat beside Philip. "But I can vote them," he said. "I am Terry Flynnt's executor. I can state unequivocally that it would be Mr. Flynnt's wish to see his son chair this meeting and I will vote accordingly."

Pennock and Whitehall put their heads together, then the lawyer said, "It doesn't matter. We expect the chairmanship of the Flynnt Group to change hands before this meeting is over. Let's get on with it."

"Very well," Philip said, "as chairman pro tem I call this extraordinary meeting of the Flynnt Group board to order. We have no pre-arranged agenda but I think the substance of the meeting is clear to us all. We're here to decide who will control this company."

"Agreed," said Pennock. The three smooth-faced money men and the old general gave their assent.

"Well," said Philip, "the success of this company under the leadership of Terry Flynnt has never been questioned. I intend to continue my father's policies. The only change I contemplate is to use a large share of my personal fortune to do good works, which will have no material effect on the company's operations. So I think it is up to those who wish to see a change in the company leadership to make their case. Mr. Pennock?"

The lawyer smiled. Something in the smile told Carras that Pennock expected that what he was about to do would be easy. "Thank you, Mr. Chairman," he said, then took a deep breath.

"Oh," said Philip, "if you'll allow me, there's one other thing."

"Please," said Pennock, "go ahead."

"Recently," said Philip, "I've come across an opportunity in the field of information technology. Very promising. But now let's hear from Mr. Pennock."

"If the board pleases, I'd like to ask Mr. Victor Whitehall to speak."

There were nods and murmurs of assent, and Whitehall took the floor. The fat man leaned back in his chair and said, "I'll make this short and blunt. I've acquired a significant position in this company's stock. It's a good company and under Terry Flynnt's leadership it would have remained a solid investment.

"But Terry Flynnt is no longer here to guide the company's affairs. Instead, his shares are going to a young man who, and I said this would be blunt, has spent his life going around in circles at a high rate of speed. Frankly, Philip Flynnt does not have the experience or the balls to run this company the way his father did. But I do. I can keep this company strong. I can keep it growing. And I can keep it in the black."

"Are you finished?" said Philip.

"Far from it," said Whitehall, "but feel free to have your say."

The young man nodded. "Gentlemen," he said, "about the worst thing you could do is to hand control of the Flynnt Group to a man, and I use the word loosely, like Victor Whitehall. A man who boarded this yacht a couple of days ago with gunmen whose orders were to kill my father and me. If it were not for Isaac Dumoulin, who was badly wounded in the fighting, we wouldn't be having this discussion today."

"If you or any of your people ever say such a thing publicly," said Arthur Pennock, "we will ruin you."

Philip made a sound of contempt. "Leaving that aside," he told the money men, "if Whitehall gets his hands on the company he will strip it of value, sell off the components and pocket most of the proceeds. You'll get a few blips on the capital gains side of the ledger, but at the cost of decades of future profits that the company could have earned for your investors."

"Hogwash," said Whitehall.

"It's what he does, gentlemen," said Philip. "Whitehall doesn't build. He devours. He'll gobble up the company and leave you nothing but the waste products of his digestion."

"Very poetic," said the fat man. He looked around the table. "All right, I've shown you the carrot. Now here's the stick. If you do not elect me to the board and give me the chairmanship of the Flynnt Group, I will dump my shares—all of them—the moment the market opens tomorrow. I calculate that a sell-off of twenty-one per cent of the company stock, coming on the heels of Terry Flynnt's death, will trigger a massive collapse of share value."

Whitehall looked at each of the mutual and pension fund managers in turn and said, "That collapse will have a significant effect on each of your portfolios. It will not look too good on your quarterly earnings statements, and it will be up to you to explain it to your masters."

Whitehall laced his fingers together and put them where his lap would have been if it wasn't covered by belly. "That's it," he said. "I'm finished."

Philip was looking tired. Carras went to him and took his wrist. The pulse was fast but strong, the old man's strong heart pounding the blood through the son's chest. "You okay?" Carras asked.

Philip's reply was a wink. He waved Carras away and spoke to the board. "If Whitehall sells tomorrow, the Flynnts will buy. And the moment the buying and selling are done, I will announce a major investment in a radical new breakthrough in artificial intelligence. Gentlemen, I have personally obtained first refusal on the prototype of a heuristic electronic circuit."

Carras saw Philip glance at Costas who was keeping a very straight face.

"A what?" said Whitehall.

"An electronic circuit that learns through trial and error," said Philip. "Not a chip that calculates and makes a mathematical determination, but a genuine synthetic brain cell. It's primitive, but it establishes the principle of a machine that can learn the way a living brain learns. That is the foundation of true artificial intelligence, the dawn of an industry that will yield not billions, but trillions of dollars in earnings over the coming decades.

"And if I am running the Flynnt Group, that breakthrough will be ours. If not, then you and your investors will have missed getting in on the ground floor of an industry that will be to the twenty-first century what automobiles were to the twentieth."

There was a silence around the table. Carras could see the fund managers running the two competing futures through the calculators that accounted for most of their mental activities. The retired general sat with his hands in his lap, waiting to see which way the meeting would go.

Whitehall spoke. "Good try, kid. Never hurts to dazzle them with shiny things and promise lots more tomorrow. But the fact is, gentlemen, even if the young man's found a goose that lays golden eggs, there's no guarantee he can keep it. Do you really want a race car driver at the wheel of a multibillion dollar corporation?"

"He'll have me to guide him," said Isaac.

Whitehall sneered. "You're just the boy's hired help, Dumoulin."

"No," said Isaac. "I'm his uncle. Terry and I were half-brothers. We ran the Flynnt Group together. There wasn't a decision these past twenty-five years that I wasn't part of."

Philip gestured to Carras who brought up an oxygen cylinder from under the young man's bed and offered him the mask so that he could take a couple of deep breaths. "That's news to me," Philip said.

"It's a long story," Isaac said. "Tell you later."

"Doesn't matter," Whitehall said. "I don't care who your daddy was, Dumoulin. You're no Terry Flynnt."

That was when the elevator doors opened and a hard voice said, "But I am."

Terry Flynnt was in a wheelchair, a mass of bandages visible through the open top of his dressing gown. Charlie Vance pushed the chair into the boardroom and placed it beside Philip's bed. He gave the room his best Jack Nicholson smile and said, "Surprise."

"Dad," said Philip. Then his eyes filled with tears.

"I didn't expect to be here either," Flynnt said. "Blame these two doctors— they put me into some kind of suspended animation and installed a nuclear powered pump in here." He tapped his bandaged chest.

"I'm so glad to see you," his son said. "I'm so sorry about all the..."

"We'll talk about it later," the older Flynnt said. "Right now you'd better let me take control of this meeting."

There were no dissents. Pennock seemed still in shock.

Flynnt looked around the table. "You'll understand why I haven't prepared any formal remarks," said the old man. "I was expecting to be somewhere else altogether, but these doctors," he indicated Carras and Vance, "took it upon themselves to keep me alive, at least for a while."

"How long will you live?" said Philip.

"Could be five minutes, could be five months," said his father. "A stroke will get me eventually. But I will spend all of that time seeing my son take full control of this corporation, so that when I finally go he and Isaac will carry on what Isaac and I have built. And God help anybody who gets in their way.

"As for the synthetic brain cell, we have already established a research institute on Forlorn Island and set aside a one billion dollar Flynnt family fund to develop the invention. You may have heard rumors about that." Flynnt turned his head sideways so that only his son and Carras saw the wink that punctuated his statement. "So, gentlemen," he concluded, "do you want a bigger and better business under the Flynnts, or do you want to eat crap from that hog of a man?"

The fund managers looked at each other. The old major general looked at his hands.

"I move that Isaac Dumoulin be elected a member of this board," Flynnt said.

"I second the motion," Philip said.

"All in favor?" Flynnt raised his hand and eyed the fund managers. The three of them put their smoothly rounded heads together and their voices were a quiet murmur. Then they straightened and three hands went up at once. The general, with a sigh of gratitude, added his to the affirmatives.

"Opposed?"

Pennock flicked his hand wearily. Whitehall glowered.

"I further move that Philip Flynnt be made chairman and chief executive officer of the Flynnt Group, and that Isaac Dumoulin be made chief operating officer with appropriate salary and benefits."

The vote was over in seconds.

"Then I think we're done here, gentlemen," said Flynnt. He looked down the table at Whitehall and added, "Now would somebody get that fat swine out of my sight?"

Whitehall's face was pale except for two bright spots of red under his slitted porcine eyes. He pushed Pennock aside and forced his way past two of the fund managers, propelling his bulk toward the elevator behind the head of the table. As he brushed past Terry Flynnt's wheelchair Flynnt said, "Good riddance."

Carras would always remember the speed with which the fat man spun. The doctor reacted, grasping for the hand that was swinging for the back of Flynnt's head—a white blur with a dark point at its center.

Whitehall was too quick. Carras's hand slid off the fabric of the fat man's sleeve. But Costas's reflexes were faster. The edge of his hand struck the assailant's wrist. Whitehall's grip flew open and something hard hit the carpeted floor with a solid thump.

Whitehall stooped to retrieve the thing that had been in his hand, but together Carras and Costas thrust the fat man into the elevator. The door closed and he was gone.

Costas bent and came up with a length of roughly shaped metal. It was a rusted and stained railroad spike.

• • •

"There's something else you have to know," Terry Flynnt said to Philip. "I killed my father."

They were all gathered in the big aft lounge, Flynnt in his wheelchair and Philip in his wheeled bed with Annabella beside him. Flynnt told again the story of that long wait on the stairs in the silent factory.

"Maybe that's why I was never much of a father to you," the old man said, "just let you grow up any old way."

There was a catch in Philip's throat. "I could have been a better son."

"No," said Flynnt, "it's up to the father to try to close the gap. I didn't try. Now there won't be much time."

Annabella put her hand on Terry's arm. "We'll make the most of it," she said.

"Still," Flynnt said, "I won't leave you with no family at all. You'll always have your uncle Isaac."

Philip said, "That was a shock. But a good one."

"I never knew he was my half-brother until his mother came to me," Flynnt said, "years after he went into the army."

She had been stricken with cancer and wanted Flynnt to know what had happened. She was ashamed of what Roddy Flynnt had done to her, but she wanted her son to know that when she died he wasn't going to be alone in the world.

"You would never take a penny of the business," Flynnt said to Isaac, "though I offered it many a time. I'm glad you're going to be there to help the boy."

"Count on it," Isaac said.

• • •

The yacht was powering back to Forlorn Island. The sea was placid and when the moon came up the water was like tarnished liquid silver.

Side by side, Athan Carras and his son leaned over the railing on the wide deck aft of the lounge. Tomorrow, the Boeing would fly them to California.

Nurse Gupta wheeled Terry Flynnt out onto the deck. Carras looked at his watch and said, "You should be resting by now."

"I'm going," Flynnt said. "I just wanted a word."

"Okay."

The old man tapped his chest. "How long do you think I've got?"

Carras shrugged. "With anti-clotting drugs, who knows?"

"I owe you for this."

"I call it even." Carras put his hand on Costas's shoulder. "You gave me back my son, the least I could do was give Philip his father."

Flynnt chuckled. "Made for an interesting board meeting."

"That was your idea."

"So I like surprising people." He looked up at the nurse. "Let's go."

"Wait," Costas said. He held out the rusted railroad spike. "Do you want this? A souvenir?"

Flynnt took the old metal and weighed it in his hand. Then he tossed it into the sea. They heard it splash in the ship's wake.

"Good night," he said.

When the old man was gone Carras looked up at the fullness of the rising moon and said, "Let me tell you about the last time I noticed that thing." He told his son about the sugar cane and the dogs and the plane and being high above the sea—and about being all alone up there.

"Truth is, I've spent the past ten years like that," Carras said. "Way up in the thin air, all alone with no idea how to get down. Didn't even know how much I needed to."

"And now?" Costas said.

"I've been lucky enough to crash and be able to walk away from it. And walk away from it is just what I intend to do."

"You're going to give up heart surgery?" Costas said. "But that's what you do. You're one of the best of the best. You save lives."

"I don't know what I'm going to do," said Carras. "That's something I've got to figure out. But this time, I'll take some advice. From you, for a start. And from your mom, if she's willing."

Epilogue

Athan and Costas Carras drove the Pantera from San Francisco to San Diego and back again, following the sometimes winding, sometimes arrow-straight Pacific Coast Highway. They got to know each other and, better than that, they got to like each other, man to man.

Carras also used the time to think. They were approaching Big Sur from the south when he came to his decision. Charlie Vance had reached him the night before on his cell phone wanting to warn him that his face was once again on front pages and television newscasts around the world.

"Terry Flynnt died of a stroke last night," he said. "And the word is out that you put his heart in his son's chest and gave him a nuclear powered one."

"Well," Carras said, "the story was bound to become public. Let Nancy Polwitz handle it."

"The media are only half of it," Vance said. "Karen Ferguson has already had two calls from wealthy men who want to know if you'll put hearts in them and ask no questions about where the organs came from. A Dr. Sturges from Wyoming has called repeatedly about a transplant."

"Wyoming? That's way outside Yale's organ procurement region."

"Sturges's daughter has cardiomyopathy; she's been waiting two years for her transplant and is deteriorating rapidly. She won't survive more than a week or two. He wants you to consider...."

"Good God," Carras said. "What have we started?"

"I imagine," Vance said, "that Pandora said pretty much the same thing."

"Pandora's box," said Carras,

"Wide open," said Vance.

So that was his legacy, or at least the part of it that most people would remember. Carras made up his mind.

When they stopped for the night at a bed and breakfast that overlooked the ocean, he gave the owners a false name and paid cash. Even so, the woman of the house looked at him as if she thought she'd seen him before.

They had dinner at a restaurant off the highway. The windows were open and they could hear the surf rolling in and out. They talked about the Flynnt Group's plans to relocate the research effort to Silicon Valley so that Costas could continue his studies at Stanford.

"You're going to be a wealthy man," Carras said.

"That's not what it's about," his son said.

"I'm glad you already know that."

The menu leaned toward grilled fish and very fresh organically grown vegetables. "Good for the heart," Costas said.

"So is this trip," his father said. He paused a moment, then said, "Do you think you would have room in your institute for a retired surgeon who wanted to do a little research? Just a corner."

"Suspended animation?" said Costas.

"That's what I'm thinking."

"I guess we could find some space."

"Good."

And that part was settled.

• • •

The Pantera's engine purred like a well-fed sabertooth as Costas wheeled the sleek car through the vine-covered gateway that led into to the Loma del Sol winery.

"Nicely handled," Athan Carras said from the passenger seat. "Park her over there."

The house was across the yard, a big old Spanish ramble of white plastered walls and age darkened beams, with red tiled roofs and steps of gray stone leading up to a wide veranda. Beth was coming out of the door as Carras levered himself out of the low slung vehicle.

"Food's ready," she said. "You're right on time." She was in jeans and a checked shirt, with her hair bound up in a cloth like Lucy in the old comedy show. To Carras she looked like a dream he thought he'd forgotten.

"No," he said, "in fact, I'm about ten years late."

She'd been reaching to remove the dust cloth from her head, but now her hand stopped halfway.

"The question is," he said, and there was something in his throat that the words had to work their way around, "is it too late?"

Costas came around from the driver's side of the car. They stood together, and anyone could have seen that they were father and son.

She removed the cloth and shook out her hair. It was long, the way she used to wear it when they were young. "We can talk about it," she said. "For now, let's just eat."

The two men walked up the stone steps and followed her into the warm aroma of her cooking. To Carras, it smelled like memories.

THE END

Technical Word Glossary

Here we briefly define some of the medical and scientific terms used in *Transplant*. You can find more complete pictures and descriptions of all aspects of heart disease and treatment in your author's other books for the general public: *Your Heart: An Owner's Guide* and *The Woman's Heart: An Owner's Guide*, both recently published by Prometheus Press.

Aortic arch

Ascending aorta

Normal Aorta

Descending aorta

Diaphragm

Abdominal aorta

Regurgitant aortic valve

Aorta—The large central artery that provides branches to supply blood to all organs of the body.

Aortic regurgitation—Leaking of blood back through the aortic valve into the left ventricle.

Arteriosclerosis—Hardening of the arteries, with accumulation of fatty deposits in the wall of the aorta.

Cardiologist—A medical doctor (not a surgeon) who specializes in diagnosis and treatment of the heart.

Cardiomyopathy—Weakening of the heart muscle. The term comes from the Greek "cardia," or heart, and "pathia," or weakness. Cardiomyopathy is called *ischemic* if it results from heart attacks or *idiopathic* if it is of unknown cause. May require a heart transplant, if prolonged and severe.

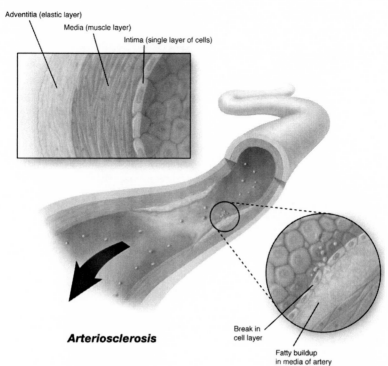

Adventitia (elastic layer)

Media (muscle layer)

Intima (single layer of cells)

Arteriosclerosis

Break in cell layer

Fatty buildup in media of artery

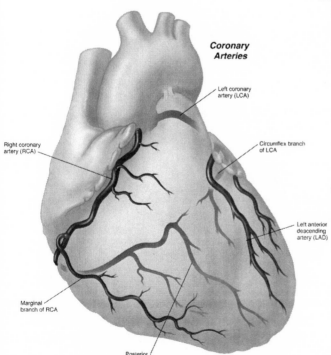

Coronary Arteries

Left coronary artery (LCA)

Right coronary artery (RCA)

Circumflex branch of LCA

Left anterior descending artery (LAD)

Marginal branch of RCA

Posterior descending branch of RCA

Coronary artery— One of the small arteries that run on the surface of the heart and provide nourishment to the heart muscle. It is the coronary arteries that become blocked and cause heart attacks.

Coumadin—A powerful blood thinning medication. Another name for this drug is Warfarin. It is used for patients with mechanical heart valves or with atrial fibrillation. Excess dosing of Coumadin can lead to catastrophic hemorrahe.

Crossmatch—Checking for compatibility between a prospective transplant recipient's blood or tissue and those of a donor.

Deep hypothermic circulatory arrest (DHCA)—A state of real-life suspended animation, in which the patient's body temperature is lowered profoundly, so that all the organs can be preserved, despite the absence of blood flow. This technique is used for complex surgery on the aorta. During DHCA, there is no pulse, no EKG, no blood pressure, no EEG (brain waves), and no blood flow; the patient is clinically dead during this interval. The patient revives when rewarmed.

Defibrillator—The paddle device used to convert serious heart rhythms to normal ones by powerful electrical discharge. As seen on TV and in the movies.

DNA—The blueprint of life—the double-helix material in the nucleus of cells that contains all our genetic material and permits reproduction.

Dobutamine—A powerful intravenous drug given to support very weak hearts. Usually given as a temporizing intervention to support a heart while awaiting an organ for transplantation.

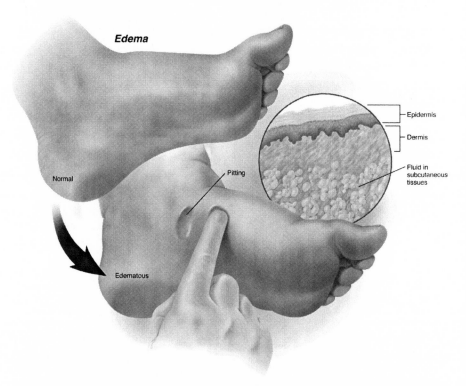

Edema—The medical term for swelling from water retention. This is usually manifested in the ankles. It can be a sign of congestive heart failure, as well as other physical problems. The edema may show an imprint if you press your finger against the swollen shin.

Exponentially—A term for describing the relationship between two phenomena.

If it is a linear relationship, the two phenomena increase in direct proportion. If it is an exponential relationship, the second phenomenon increases faster than the first, increasing to the second or third power, or the like, while the first phenomenon simply doubles. The metabolic rate decreases exponentially as the body temperature falls.

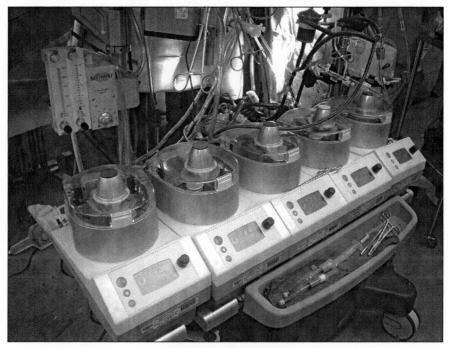

Heart-lung machine

Heart-lung machine—The mechanical device that takes over the functions of the heart and the lungs while the most intricate segments of open heart surgery are performed. It includes a pump to circulate the blood and an artificial lung. The heart-lung machine is colloquially called, in professional circles, simply, "the pump."

Left atrium—The upper left chamber of the heart, which receives blood from the lungs and passes the blood on to the powerful left ventricle.

Left ventricle—The powerful left lower chamber of the heart, which supplies blood to all parts of the body.

Lidocaine—A powerful "anti-arrhythmic" medication, used to correct the very serious abnormal rhythms called ventricular tachycardia and ventricular fibrillation.

Lymph node—One of the "glands" of the body, which are found in the neck and groin regions, among other locations. These important structures, usually about the size of a kidney bean, can be sampled from a prospective donor. They are then put into a test tube with the prospective recipient's blood. If they do not react, then the transplant can be performed safely, without fear of rejection. This preliminary matching test has been termed, appropriately, a "transplant in a bottle."

Nucleus—The center, or heart, of a cell, which contains the genetic material essential for reproduction.

Pericardium—The thin, glistening, flexible but inelastic (nonstretchable) sac that surrounds the heart in its central position in the chest.

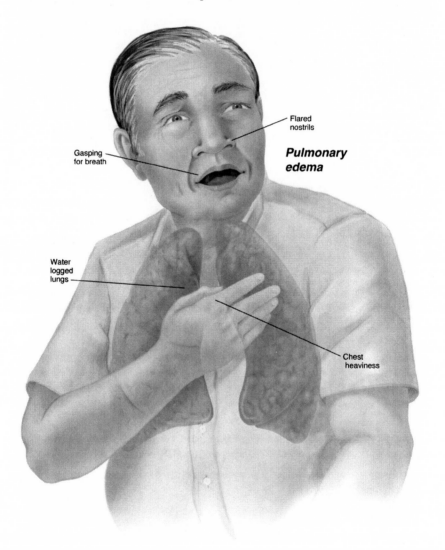

Pulmonary edema—A state of flooding of the lungs with fluid backed up behind a weak heart. Shortness of breath is usually profound. This is a very serious manifestation of congestive heart failure.

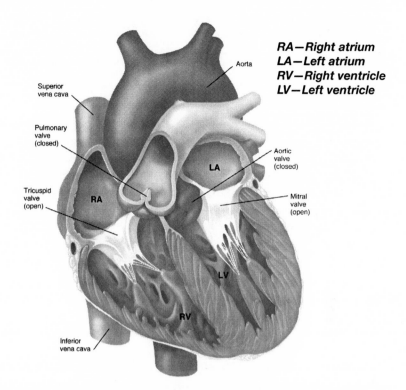

RA—*Right atrium*
LA—*Left atrium*
RV—*Right ventricle*
LV—*Left ventricle*

Aorta

Superior vena cava

Pulmonary valve (closed)

Aortic valve (closed)

LA

Tricuspid valve (open)

RA

Mitral valve (open)

LV

RV

Inferior vena cava

Right atrium—The upper chamber of the right side of the heart, responsible for receiving the spent blood from the body and delivering it to the right ventricle.

Right ventricle—The powerful lower chamber of the right side of the heart, which delivers the blood to the lungs.

Pathogens—Bacteria or viruses causing human disease.

Solumedrol—A powerful steroid medication, used to suppress rejection after a transplant. This drug must be given intravenously at the time of a heart transplant, in order to prevent immediate rejection of the transplanted organ.

Steroid—A family of powerful anti-rejection drugs. Prednisone is one oral form and Solumedrol is one intravenous form.

Tissue typing—Laboratory testing to determine if a prospective transplant donor and recipient are immunologically compatible.

Figures in Glossary © John A. Elefteriades 2008.

Ethical issues in *Transplant*
Author's discussion questions

This novel makes us consider multiple conflicts regarding life patterns and decisions. Can one devastate one's family relationships—wife, children, marriage—in a quest for professional success? Is such a serious situation ever recoverable? Can people really grow, appreciate their shortcomings, and restore meaning to lost relationships? Is it right for a formerly hot but now aging actress to seduce a susceptible surgeon under false pretenses, in order to win a movie role for herself? Is this not truly a victimless crime? We ponder these heady non-medical issues as we watch Carras, Costas, and Beth, as well as Flynnt and Philip, and Hilary as well, struggle and grow.

The heart of this novel, however, has to do with ethical issues in contemporary medicine. When is the right time to take an experimental procedure to clinical application in human beings? Is it right to expose the first patient or patients to an untried technique? Is not the entire history of medicine and surgery one of brave surgeons and patients navigating their way through uncharted waters. What alternative is there? How else can medicine advance?

Beyond those issues, the single key ethical issue raised in this novel has to do with whether a father has the right to give his own heart to save his son.

Magazines and newspapers are full of laudatory stories about mothers, fathers, brothers, sisters, and more distant relatives selflessly giving their organs to a family member. There is no question that an organ from a related individual is a much better immunologic "match" than an organ from a stranger—leading to better long-term results. As in our novel, the situation often does arise in which a needy recipient is unknowingly "immunized" (or, rendered allergic) in the course of daily life to organs from unrelated individuals. This acquired allergy to the tissues of strangers usually does not apply to tissues from family members. Donations from family members usually match very well, immunologically. We view organ donations from family members as a wonderful expression of human love.

In many cases, even an unrelated individual donates an organ for a stranger. Again, magazines and newspapers are replete with tales of such totally selfless acts of kindness to one's fellow man. This is, after all, what the Bible preaches. Jesus says very clearly, in John 15, *Greater love hath no man than this, that a man lay down his life for his friends*. If one can lay down his life for a friend, then certainly even more so for one's child.

The scenario in the present novel is different from any faced up to now in the real world. The difference resides in the fact that the heart is an unpaired organ. We have only one heart. We have two kidneys, two lungs, and liver that can be divided into multiple lobes. A kidney donor, a lung donor, or a partial liver donor has every expectation to live a normal life (although he does face a low, but real, possibility of complication or even death from the donor operation). A heart donor—if there ever should be one— is certain to die immediately upon donation. Herein arises the core ethical dilemma in this novel.

The idea of giving one's life for another has a long and honored history. The ancient Greek playwright Euripides presented this scenario in *Alcestis;* the heroine for whom the play is named gave her life so that her husband could live (eternally). The Bible condones such ultimate sacrifice as an expression of love for one's fellow man. Yet, when we think of the father, Flynnt, forcing the surgeon, Carras, to take his heart out and place it in another human being, we cringe. Why?

Please ponder the following specific ethical questions arising from the key conflict in this novel:

1. Just a few short months ago, the world was captivated by a news report about a marine in Iraq who saw a grenade come through the hatch and land on the floor of his armored vehicle. The marine deliberately threw himself onto the grenade, condemning himself to instantaneous death, but saving the lives of the four comrades riding in the tank with him. Society views this as an ultimate expression of heroism. The marine received a posthumous award for his bravery. Why is this marine a hero and Flynnt an ogre? Is it not inherent in the very concept of war that some will give their lives for others, whom they do not even know?

2. If Flynnt wants to give his life and his heart, why should Carras not be allowed or even encouraged to carry out the operation? Why should such a decision not be within the scope of human freedoms? How much responsibility falls on Flynnt and how much on Carras?

3. Would you get in the way of a bullet headed for your son or daughter? I would, without thinking. How is this different from Flynnt's giving his life for his son? Is there something different because Flynnt's actions are deliberate, calculated, and executed over months, as opposed to suddenly and reflexively stopping a flying bullet?

4. Flynnt threatens Carras's own son, Costas. Would Carras be justified in performing the forbidden transplant in order to spare his own son's life? Why should Carras even hesitate—thereby jeopardizing the life of an innocent young man, his own son, no less, when Flynnt willingly insists on donating his own heart? And, after all, Flynnt's desired donation is for Flynnt's very own son.

5. How does the reader think that Phillip will feel about his own continuing to live as a consequence of his father's sacrifice of his life? In Alcestis, the husband was overwhelmed and incapacitated by his wife's selfless donation. Will Phillip be able to live with this? How will the events in this novel affect Phillip's prior near-loathing of his father?

6. As far as your author is aware, no one in history has ever donated his own heart to a loved one for transplantation. The news media have made presentations about the black market in organs—mainly kidneys. But, these are unwilling donors whose organs are stolen. It has been documented, as well, that poor individuals have sold a kidney for money for their families (almost never producing any substantive sustained improvement in the family financial situation). We are not aware of a single heart ever being sold with similar intent. Nor are we aware—yet—of a single willing donation of one's own heart. Do you think that the mere publication of this novel will encourage this type of self-sacrifice? Will we really get calls from mothers and fathers wanting to donate for their children?

7. Say that this novel does open Pandora's box—as Carras and Vance find to be the case. Is your author ethically responsible for facilitating the opening of Pandora's box by virtue of the very act of writing this novel?

Ethical issues in *Transplant*
Dr. Baillie's discussion questions

Dr. Harold Baillie, Provost and Professor of Philosophy at the University of Scranton, is a foremost authority on the ethics of medicine. He has written a respected textbook for college courses entitled Health Care Ethics, *now in its Second Edition.*

Respect for life is the foundation of medical ethics. It is the root of the Hippocratic Oath and the reason why that oath has retained its power for much longer than two millennia. While a concern with medical ethics is obviously quite ancient, there has been a recent resurgence of interest that began in the late nineteen-fifties with the development of kidney dialysis machines. Initially, the interest was forced by the limited availability of the dialysis machines; respect for life required an ethical basis for decisions regarding who would be treated by dialysis and who would not. This often meant deciding who would live and who would die.

A simple solution to this problem involved more production of machines, and for a while the development of new medical technologies was closely enough matched by increases in production that it appeared that this type of medical ethics issue would disappear. In its place, the discussion of the ethics of practicing medicine shifted to concerns with patient autonomy and the right of the patient to provide informed consent. What began as a concern with the physician gaining the patient's permission to touch the patient quickly became a complex discussion of the extent of patient autonomy and the responsibilities of the physician (or any other health care giver) to follow or to limit the patient's decision-making, whether because of the physician's medical knowledge or personal ethics.

Along with the discussion of medical ethics, there has been a discussion of the ethics of scientific research. There are many different types of scientific research, but medical research, like medical practice, finds its ethical core in respect for human life. Scientific research typically looks for results that are confirmed by repetition and fit into the known system of science. To protect human life, medical research relies on ideas that may originate in a laboratory experiment, but then move on to extensive animal testing. Only after the research suggests strong positive results is the procedure carefully tested on humans, first in small numbers, and then in larger; each step of the way is characterized by intense analysis of the results. The goal is to identify and minimize any risk to human patients, yet also to confirm the medical benefit to a patient.

Today, we are well aware of how complex discussions of the ethics of both medical practice and medical research have become, and it is this complexity that is so well presented in Dr. Elefteriades' book. Early in the book, Carras' willingness to operate on Dr. Goldenberg is the reason for the original attacks on Carras' character. He appears to have violated the ethics of medical research by rushing from incomplete animal testing (and the lack of support from the research ethics committee) to human use of the procedure. There is a clear tension between Carras' desire to save the life of his friend and the need to protect human life by patiently investigating the variety of potential consequences of the new and radical surgical procedure. Does Dr. Goldenberg's imminent death relieve Carras of the ethical obligation to proceed cautiously? Can we experiment on those we are reasonably certain will die soon, or must we respect their humanity by remaining cautious? As another example, Terry's nuclear powered heart pump produces clots, one of which eventually kills him. It does not matter how many pumps we produce, there remains the unsolved research problem of those clots.

Technology has limits beyond our capacity for production. In its own way, supply remains a problem. The heart transplant that Philip needs requires an available and compatible human organ, and the supply of a heart with the needed tissue type is virtually non-existent. Terry's willingness to die in order to supply a heart for his son provides a practical solution to the supply problem, but it raises serious questions about the range of Terry's autonomy. Can a patient arrange to die in order to provide an organ for transplant? Do we own our body in such a way that we can distribute its "parts" at our will?

But Terry's desire to provide his own heart to heal Philip requires the cooperation of Dr. Carras. Even if Terry has the right to dispose of his own heart, does he have the right to require Carras to perform the surgery? Carras' personal ethics (as well as the laws of the United States and the strictures of even the Hippocratic Oath) loudly proclaim that this act of killing one in order to save the other cannot be done. Ordinarily, this would settle the question. But Terry tries first to bribe Carras and later to force him into submission through kidnapping and torture. Terry's assumption that every man has his price fails in the face of Carras' ethical convictions.

One can follow Carras and conclude that Terry is unethical and coercive, deserving to be completely frustrated in his efforts to force the doctor to operate. The nagging problem permeating this book, however, is not so easily resolved. Is Terry's desperate attempt to save his son, even to the extent of using his massive economic resources in ethically despicable ways, truly wrong? This is not simply a question of balancing a hierarchy of ethical principles, the task of weighing the good and the bad, or even simply recognizing the good and separating it from the bad. This is about the life of Terry's son, literally a question of flesh and blood. Can one be said to truly respect life if one cannot save one's own flesh and blood, given the opportunity? Would Terry be ethical if he (arguably, selfishly) refused to give up his heart while his son died from the lack of a transplant?

Carras, of course, initially argues that the issue is suicide and murder, not self-sacrifice. From this perspective, Terry is trying to commit suicide, and in order to do so, is trying to force Carras to murder him. As a matter of principle, this interpretation of circumstances makes sense. However, Terry, and eventually Vance, argues that Carras is not addressing the true ethical issues. They suggest that Carras is simply "trying to win," reacting to a deep seated, perhaps unconscious, desire to control all around him. In other words, they suggest that Carras' ethics is nothing more than selfishness, an inability emotionally to open to other people hidden in an effort to dominate others. Carras' own family problems, including his non-extistent relationship with his son, are cited as evidence of this selfishness.

This final argument of the book raises deep questions about the nature and origin of ethics. Where do our ethics principles come from? Are they rational, expressing our ability to think in universal terms that transcend the personal? Much of ethical thought rests on this assumption, expressed by leading historical figures like Kant or a contemporary medical ethician such as Norman Daniels. Or are they, rather, expressions of what is most personal about us? Nietzsche argued that an individual's ethics is simply the expression of her or his psychological make-up. What one thinks is right or wrong is the result of how one's will is shaped by one's personal history. For example, the commitment to one another that Terry and Isaac share seems rooted in their family history, while Maigrot seems to choose right or wrong out of a fear of physical harm that has roots in his childhood.

The enjoyment to be found in this book is rooted in its ability to raise profound ethical questions in the very practical (if somewhat fantastical) situations of an action novel.

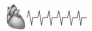

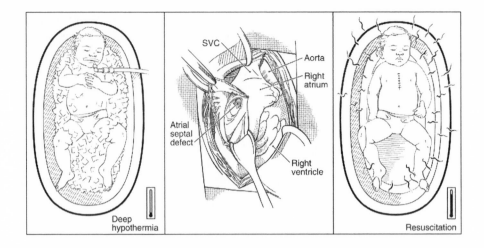

SVC

Aorta

Right atrium

Atrial septal defect

Right ventricle

Deep hypothermia

Resuscitation

Real-life clinical application
of suspended animation in cardiac surgery

Real-life suspended animation is applied daily at our hospital and many others throughout the world.

This technique was originally begun in babies with "a hole in the heart." In the fifties and early sixties, before the heart-lung machine became available, daring surgeons put babies into an ice bath until their hearts stopped. The cold temperature protected the children's internal organs while the surgeons put the baby on an operating table, quickly opened the chest, and placed a stitch to close the hole in the heart. They then closed the incision quickly and re-warmed the baby in a hot water bath. As the baby warmed, the heart restarted, and the patient awakened to a normal life, forever cured of the "hole" in the heart and its otherwise debilitating or life-threatening consequences.

The figures on this page illustrate how this immersion technique was clinically practiced, allegedly originating in the Siberian regions of Russia— where cold was abundant and easily tapped for medical application.

Today, we use hypothermia routinely for complex surgery on the aortic arch, the part of the aorta that gives off branches to the arms and the brain. (See the figure of the aorta in the Glossary.) We produce real-life suspended animation at a temperature of 18°C (or 64°F). During this time, we shut off the heart lung machine—and the patient is without EKG (electrocardiogram, or heart wave trace), EEG (electroencephalogram, or brain wave trace), pulse, blood pressure, or blood flow. In other words, there are absolutely no signs of life. We can sustain this state nearly invariably safely for 45 minutes, and usually safely for 60 minutes. Cold is remarkably protective of biological tissues. The metabolic rate falls as temperature decreases—meaning that very little blood flow is required to keep an organ alive at low temperatures. The drop in metabolic rate is not linear, but rather, exponential; that means that the metabolic rate falls much more rapidly than the temperature decreases. In other words, hypothermia is very, very protective. The patients undergoing aortic surgery via this technique awaken normally, with fully restored cognitive function—memories, abilites, instincts, etc. We often find the patients reading their favorite novels or magazines by evening of the same day.

The fact that patients do so well, with all their cognitive functions, memories, skills, instincts, and talents intact, leads me to surmise that storage of information in the brain must be "hard-wired" is some way, so that the relevant "connections" are preserved even without energy (blood flow).

The paper cited below chronicles, in a presentation to our cardiac surgical society, your author's experience with this technique in nearly 400 human patients. Since the publication of this report, your author has treated hundreds of additional patients in this way. The scientific report is intended to document the safety of what we call straight (ie. unaugmented) *deep hypothermic circulatory arrest*, or "DHCA" for short.

Straight Deep Hypothermic Arrest: Experience in 394 Patients Supports Its Effectiveness as a Sole Means of Brain Preservation

Presented at the Forty-third Annual Meeting of The Society of Thoracic Surgeons, San Diego, CA, Jan. 29–31, 2007.

Arjet Gega MD[a], John A. Rizzo PhD[c, d], Michele H. Johnson MD[b], Maryann Tranquilli RN[a], Emily A. Farkas MD[a] and John A. Elefteriades MD[a], [a]Section of Cardiothoracic Surgery, Yale University School of Medicine, New Haven, Connecticut [b]Department of Diagnostic Imaging, Yale University School of Medicine, New Haven, Connecticut [c]Department of Preventive Medicine, State University of New York, Stony Brook, Stony Brook, New York [d]Department of Economics, State University of New York, Stony Brook, Stony Brook, New York

Background

The three methods of brain preservation for aortic arch surgery—straight deep hypothermic circulatory arrest (DHCA) without perfusion adjuncts, retrograde cerebral perfusion, and antegrade cerebral perfusion—remain controversial. Patients in this report underwent surgery solely with DHCA.

Methods

Straight DHCA at 19°C was used in 394 patients (267 males, 127 females) during a 10-year period. Mean age was 61.3 years (range, 15 to 88 years). Eighty-seven cases (22.1%) were urgent or emergencies. Thirty-eight (9.6%) were performed for descending or thoracoabdominal pathology and the rest for ascending/arch (102 hemiarch, 49 total arch). Ninety-one patients (23.1%) had dissections. The head was packed in ice. No barbiturate coma was used.

Results

DHCA lasted a mean of 31.0 minutes (range, 10 to 66 minutes). Reexploration for bleeding was required in 4.5% (18/394). Overall mortality was 6.3% (25/394). Mortality was 3.6% (11/307) for elective cases and 16% (14/87) for emergency cases. The stroke rate was 4.8% (19/394). The seizure rate was 3.1% (12/394). Forty-five patients with high professional cognitive demands (MD, PhD, attorney, etc) performed without detriment postoperatively. Among patients with DHCA exceeding 40 minutes, the stroke rate was 13.1% (8/61); a neuroradiologist's review of brain computed tomography scans found 62.5% of these strokes (5/8) to be embolic and 37.5% (3/8) hypoperfusion related. By multivariable logistic regression, emergency operation and descending location increased morbidity and mortality.

Conclusions

Straight DHCA without adjunctive perfusion suffices as a sole means of cerebral protection. Stroke and seizure rates are low. Cognitive function, by clinical assessment, is excellent. Especially for straightforward ascending/arch reconstructions, there is little need for the added complexity of brain perfusion strategies.

The following article is reprinted with permission from the New Haven (Conn.) Register:

Woman who was declared dead thaws, is revived after several hours

Sunday, February 19, 2006 3:00 AM EST
By Abram Katz

Her breathing, brain waves and pulse stopped for about six to eight hours. Penelope has no recollection of the missing period. It was just an unconscious blank. One moment she was alive. Then she was in a hospital.

"Right now, I feel great. I didn't know I was dead," she said days after the unusual incident.

But her husband remembers all too well.

He found her on an unheated porch in the predawn darkness of a frigid day in January. The temperature was 14 or 15 degrees.

Her eyes were open and fixed, her skin pale and cold, her heart still and lungs silent.

"When I found my wife with her eyes open — that vision will stay with me. I heard her gasp, so I thought she was breathing," he said. But it was a death rattle.

Penelope is fine now, except for tingling in her feet and arms, probably the result of slight frostbite.

Doctors marvel at her recovery.

She was declared dead and given up for dead at a clinic before she somehow blossomed back to life at Yale-New Haven Hospital.

Dr. Lawrence McChesney, trauma surgeon at Yale-New Haven, was less than optimistic when her body arrived by LifeStar helicopter.

He saw her the next day when she was warm, had a pulse and brain waves and was breathing.

"You look really good for a dead lady," McChesney quipped.

Penelope inadvertently cooled her body into a state of "suspended animation" similar to the condition that cardiothoracic surgeons call "deep hypothermic circulatory arrest."

Penelope apparently chilled just the right way and was rescued literally minutes before her death became permanent, physicians and surgeons said.

Dr. John A. Elefteriades, chief of cardiothoracic surgery at Yale-New Haven, said patients are routinely chilled before aortic surgery.

Surgeons cool the patient's core temperature to about 66 degrees. The heart and brain stop all by themselves.

With no blood flow, clamps can be removed, giving surgeons access to parts of the aorta that must be repaired, Elefteriades said.

"Patients can't stay without circulation indefinitely. The brain needs oxygen. Forty-five minutes is OK, and 60 minutes is usually safe. After that, brain cells start dying," he said.

Elefteriades was finishing a heart transplant in an adjacent operating room when Penelope concluded her medical voyage from a local clinic to Yale-New Haven.

"She was found at just the right time. I think she was very lucky. Basically, it's a miracle," he said.

Penelope's husband, Stan, said the couple had been out with friends.

Penelope apparently had a few cocktails, doctors said.

Stan went upstairs to bed. Penelope went to retrieve something from the car.

"Then I woke up in the hospital," she said.

Stan said he was awakened by the couple's two dogs at about 5 a.m. and went looking for his wife.

"They love their mom. They knew something was wrong," he said.

"I found Penelope, her eyes wide open. I threw warm water in her face, wrapped her in a blanket and called 911." He pinched her, hoping the minor pain would bring her back to consciousness. No response.

She gasped, but that was probably her last breath, Stan said.

Emergency medical technicians loaded Penelope into an ambulance. One radioed ahead to the hospital, reporting that the patient was dead, Stan said. As the ambulance proceeded to a Shoreline medical center the EMT summoned a LifeStar helicopter.

"They worked on her for two hours. Then the doctor came out and said 'I'm sorry,'" Stan said.

Meanwhile, the helicopter had arrived and the medical center was sending it back empty, when a nurse heard a lone beep from one of the instruments monitoring Penelope.

"She has a pulse!" the woman shouted.

Fortunately, the helicopter was still preparing to leave. Penelope was placed on board and whisked to the landing pad at Yale-New Haven.

"The first question was, 'Is it worth going ahead?'" Elefteriades said. "I said 'Yes.'"

"We put in lines. There was no pulse," McChesney said.

"Warming her from the outside would be useless," he said, so catheters were placed in her femoral vein and artery and circulated through a machine that oxygenated and warmed her blood.

"She came in at 80 degrees. At 86 degrees, Penelope's heart stirred. As the temperature rose, it started to beat, and at an internal temperature of about 99, her heart started to actually pump blood and her kidneys began making urine.

"I was extremely surprised. The next day, she was talking and behaving normally. I thought her brain would be injured. I thought at best she would be brain dead," McChesney said.

"I remember going out my door. Then I woke up and saw my brother and everyone else," Penelope said.

"Nothing hurt except the tube down my throat. My feet were numb and my arms were tingling," she said.

"I appreciate life more. I'm just grateful to everyone," she said.

Elefteriades said Penelope probably survived because she cooled very slowly over several hours.

"She was cooling from the external environment. She slowed down like a hibernating animal," he said.

Elefteriades said the technique of cooling surgical patients was developed in Siberia to repair heart defects in babies. The infant would be placed in ice water. An abnormality would be fixed with a stitch or two, the incision would be closed and the tiny patient placed in a bath of warm water.

After Penelope was clearly out of danger, doctors were pondering the many implications of her strange experience.

"I wonder if she could collect on her life insurance. She was dead," a physician said.

....

The following article is reprinted with permission from the New York Times:

Daring rescue in frigid river saves 8-year-old

Published: January 21, 1987
By DENNIS HEVESI

A former New Haven police officer and a New York City firefighter were credited yesterday with a daring rescue in which they pulled an 8-year-old boy from a submerged van that was being dragged into the frigid currents of a Connecticut river.

The boy's mother died of heart failure after the accident. But his father, brother and sister — considered "basically dead" when brought to Yale-New Haven Hospital — were revived by more than 40 members of the hospital staff who formed three cardio-pulmonary teams.

By yesterday afternoon, the brother and sister had regained consciousness. The father was listed in extremely critical condition, according to a hospital spokesman, Glenda Bethune.

A spokesman for the Connecticut State Police, Sgt. Daniel Lewis, said the accident took place at 3:42 P.M. Monday, in the westbound lanes of Interstate 95, near the town line between Madison and Guilford, Conn.

Van Becomes Submerged

"The highway was very icy," Sergeant Lewis said, "and the van vaulted over the cables and landed in the East River," which flows south into the Long Island Sound.

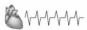

"The entire van was submerged about 25 feet from the shore," he said. "There was about 18 inches of water running over the top of the van."

The former police officer, 39-year-old Robert Ramadei of Northford, Conn., said he was driving home when he saw the yellow van, driven by Cesar A. Alvarez, 40, of 132 Guy Lombardo Avenue, Freeport, L.I., "spin out of control and crash through the cable." It was Mr. Alvarez's son, Cesar D. Alvarez, that Mr. Ramadei and the firefighter, Barry Meade, 37, of Port Washington, L.I., are credited with saving.

Mr. Ramadei said he ran down the embankment but by the time he got near the van, the current was taking it further into the river. "I could hear the people screaming and I knew there were children in there," he said.

Grabbing an Ankle

Mr. Ramadei swam out to the van. "The vehicle was totally submerged," he said. "I dove down to the passenger door and I could not open it. The terrifying thing was that I could see the people and they were in a total panic situation. I swam to the driver's door. I was unsuccessful in opening that door.

"I then swam to the top of the van, which was 18 inches under water. There was one of these crank-open vents. I smashed that with my hand. I had to submerge my right arm and head to reach in and feel around. The interior was full of debris. Thank God, I came up with Cesar's ankle. And I pulled him through by his ankle."

By then, Mr. Meade, a scuba diver with the City Fire Department's Rescue Co. 1 in Manhattan, had swam to the van with ropes from his car. "I reached into the van and tried to find anyone else I could reach," Mr. Meade said. "but the hole wasn't big enough.

"The child wasn't breathing," he said. "Bob gave him some back compressions, and the child cried. He mumbled, 'Mommy, Daddy.' "

With the rope, Mr. Meade said he tied Mr. Ramadei and the boy together. "Bob swam the child to shore," with people on the shore pulling them in," he said. "I only wish we could have gotten the rest of the family out."

Sergeant Lewis said emergency crews managed to secure the van with cables. "They had people in cold-water survival suits," he said "By breaking out one of the windows, they reached inside and pulled out three more people" — Carmen Alvarez, 32; her son, Mark, 12, and daughter, Isalia, 4. Later, a state trooper found the father.

Mrs. Alvarez was pronounced dead at 7:51 P.M. at St. Raphael's Hospital in New Haven. But at Yale-New Haven, Dr. John E. Fenn said that medical teams managed to restore the heartbeats of Mr. Alvarez, Mark and Isalia. "These people arrived basically dead," Dr. Fenn said. "No pulse, no blood pressures, no respiration. Their temperatures were approxmately 73 degrees."

Sergeant Lewis said Mr. Ramadei and Mr. Meade "really took a chance."

"It only takes a few minutes in waters of that temperature when you're not equipped with cold-water gear to lose control of your own muscles," he said. "They certainly are heroes."

The heart-and-a-half operation is real

Your author and his team really are exploring the "heart-and-a-half" option for heart transplantation. The potential benefits of this novel technique, currently in the final preclinical stages of laboratory investigation, are described accurately in the early chapters of this novel.

The news article reproduced below summarizes, for a general audience, the principles involved in this novel method of transplantation. This article, reporting our technique for a general audience, followed our publication of multiple scientific reports on this technique. We hope to proceed to clinical application in human patients in the near future.

The determination of when a novel operation has been investigated sufficiently to permit human application raises all sorts of ethical issues, none of which have ever been fully resolved.

....

The following article is reprinted with permission from Yale Scientific Magazine 77.3 Spring 2004:

Something Old, Something New

Imagine two people who lift at the gym. One curls ten pounds while the other curls forty. With time, the one who curls forty builds up stronger arm muscles than the other. What would happen if you suddenly tell the weaker person to curl forty pounds? He simply would not be able to. "The same is true with heart transplantation," describes cardiothoracic surgeon Dr. John Elefteriades, Chief of the Section of Cardiothoraric Surgery. Heart attacks usually occur in the left ventricle, which gradually fails. As a result, blood backs up in the lungs, causing pulmonary edema – fluid buildup – and hypertension. Unlike the weakening left ventricle, the right ventricle becomes hypertrophic as its muscles enlarge over time to pump blood against higher pulmonary pressure. This condition leads to congestive heart failure and the need for a new heart. After transplantation, however, the patient faces a different problem: the right ventricle of the donor heart is not strong enough to pump blood through the patient's lungs, much like the habitual ten-pound lifter who is not strong enough to lift forty pounds.

In right ventricle-sparing heart transplantation, a "heart an a half" is created by joining the right half of the receipient's heart to a full donor heart. (Credit: John Elefteriades)

To overcome donor heart failure, Elefteriades and fellow Yale collaborators developed right ventricle-sparing heart transplantation, also known as the "heart and a half" procedure, where only the left half of the patient's heart is removed and the right half is attached to a full donor heart. The result of one and a half hearts has both a functional left ventricle and a strong right one. This procedure, however, introduces a host of vexing problems. Because the heart is one big muscle with no planes of division, it is difficult to separate the two halves without disrupting its electrical and vascular system or causing over-bleeding, and after separation, all the correct connections between donor and patient heart must be made. Since 2000, Elefteriades' team has already moved the procedure into the last pre-clinical stage of testing.

Permissions

Cover photo: Courtesy of Robert A. Lisak © 2008
Photo of heart-lung machine on page 237: John A. Elefteriades © 2008
New Haven Register
New York Times
Yale Scientific Magazine
Photo of Dr. Elefteriades on page 256: John A. Elefteriades © 2008
Jet airplane on back cover: With permission and © 2008 Sascha Burkard

Acknowledgments

Thanks go first and foremost to Matt Hughes, the brilliant author of science fiction books including *Fools Errant* and *Fool Me Twice*, whose skills enhanced the original manuscript of *Transplant* immeasurably.

A special thank you goes to Dr. Harold (Hal) Baillie, Professor of Ethics and Provost of the University of Scranton, for his insightful ethical commentary, which appears in the didactic Back Matters of this book. Dr.Baillie has authored the respected and popular textbook *Healthcare Ethics*, now in its Second Edition.

Heartfelt thanks go to Robot Binaries and Press and to Publisher Dr. Howard S. Smith, author of *I, robot*, who had faith in a first-time novelist and who personally shepherded this book into its present form, and Kathy Harestad for the cover, layout and typesetting.

Cover photo courtesy of Robert A. Lisak © 2008

Many thanks to readers

We thank you for reading our story and perusing the didactic materials in the Back Matter. We hope that we have entertained you, informed you painlessly about certain medical concepts, and, especially, involved you in contemplating some important ethical issues in modern medicine, and transplantation in particular. Your feelings about our characters and the ethical issues involved are important to us. We welcome you to visit our *Transplant* website (www.robotpress.net) and to write us your comments about these matters.

Thank you.

John A. Elefteriades, MD

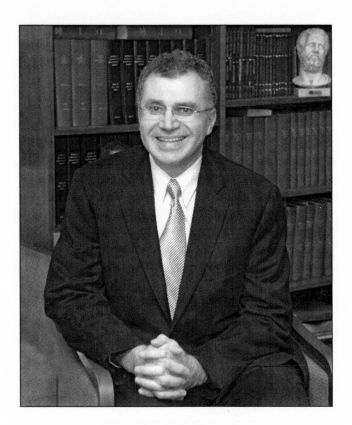

About the Author

John A. Elefteriades, MD

Dr. John Elefteriades is the William W.L. Glenn Professor of Cardiothoracic Surgery and Chief of Cardiac Surgery at Yale University and Yale New-Haven Hospital. He is among the most clinically active academic surgeons in the country.

Dr. Elefteriades graduated magna cum laude with a triple major in Physics, French and Psychology from Yale University. He received his MD degree from the Yale University School of Medicine. He trained at Yale in both general surgery and cardiothoracic surgery. After completing his training, he joined the faculty at the Yale University School of Medicine.

He performs all aspects of adult cardiac and thoracic surgery. He is a recognized authority in interventions for the failing left ventricle, including coronary artery bypass grafting, left ventricular aneurysmectomy, and artificial heart implantation. Dr. Elefteriades directs the Center of Thoracic Aortic Disease at Yale, one of the nation's largest facilities for treatment of the dilated thoracic aorta. He conducts laboratory research in new techniques of heart transplantation and aortic surgery. Among his research projects, he is working with Celera Diagnostics to identify the genetic mutations responsible for thoracic aortic aneurysms.

Dr. Elefteriades serves on multiple scientific advisory and editorial boards. He is a past President of the Connecticut Chapter of the American College of Cardiology and

 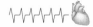

member of the national Board of Governors of the College. Dr. Elefteriades is also past President of the International College of Angiology. He serves on the editorial board of the *American Journal of Cardiology, the Journal of Cardiac Surgery, Cardiology, and the Journal of Thoracic and Cardiovascular Surgery.* He is a member of the Thoracic Surgery Director's Association and has been named consistently in The Best Doctors in America. He is a frequently requested international lecturer, visiting professor and guest surgeon. He is the author of over 200 scientific publications on a wide range of cardiac and thoracic topics. He was selected as one of the ten best doctors in America by *Men's Health* magazine. He has been featured in many dozens of print, radio, and television presentations. He has been awarded the Walter Bleifeld Memorial Award for Distinguished Contribution in Clinical Research in Cardiology and the John B. Chang Research Achievement Award. In 2005 he was selected to lecture at the Leadership in Biomedicine Series at the Yale University School of Medicine. In 2006, he received the Socrates Award from the Thoracic Residents Association, Thoracic Surgery Directors' Association, and the Society of Thoracic Surgeons, recognizing exceptional achievement in teaching and mentorship of residents. In 2007, together with the Yale Office of Cooperative Research, Dr. Elefteriades started CoolSpine, to pursue novel mechanisms for spinal cord and brain protection. This work is being supported by the National Science Foundation.

Dr. Elefteriades was named the William W.L. Glenn Professor of Cardiothoracic Surgery in 2006. This endowed chair honors the memory of Dr. Elefteriades' mentor, Dr. Glenn. Dr. Elefteriades is the author of the books *House Officer Guide to ICU Care (1st and 2nd Editions), Advanced Treatment Options for the Failing Left Ventricle, Diseases of the Aorta, Your Heart: An Owner's Guide, The Woman's Heart: An Owner's Guide,* and *Acute Aortic Disease.*